Contents

Introduction

If you've just learned that you have a cataract, you may be apprehensive about what happens next. Rest assured, cataracts are a very common eye problem, typically related to normal aging. We're all likely to experience cataracts—the clouding of the eye's lens. Fortunately, the vast majority of people who suffer from cataracts today can undergo successful outpatient surgery to treat them. In many cases, physicians can remove the cataracts and improve vision problems such as nearsightedness, farsightedness, or even astigmatism.

As cataract surgeons, we want to help our patients make informed decision about their cataract treatment. We wrote this book to help you understand how cataracts are removed and how your visual clarity is restored. We explain advances in technology and techniques that have made cataract surgery the most commonly performed operation in the United States. We hope that *Cataract Surgery* educates you about how cataracts are removed as well as give you peace of mind about your surgical procedure.

1

Cataracts: An Overview

Age-related cataracts are common. Most of us will develop them as we grow older. The American Academy of Ophthalmology suggests that by age seventy-five, 70 percent of adult Americans will experience the blurring and distorted vision associated with cataracts. Statistics suggest that by the year 2020, cataracts will affect more than 30 million Americans, a considerably higher number than the 20 million adults affected today.

But what exactly is a cataract? What are the symptoms? And what puts you at risk for developing them? It's important that you pay attention to cataracts once they start developing because they can gradually, but significantly, reduce your vision and even cause blindness. The good news is that, thanks to modern medicine, cataracts are very treatable, and impaired vision can be restored.

What Is a Cataract?

The term *cataract* has ancient roots in the Greek and Latin terms for "waterfall." That's because centuries ago people believed the clouding in their eyes actually came from an opaque material flowing like water over their eyes. Indeed, a cataract is a clouding of the eye lens. As the cloudiness increases, the cataract can blur or distort your vision and cause colors to fade. If not treated, cataracts can lead to blindness. Most cataracts are related to

Eye Anatomy

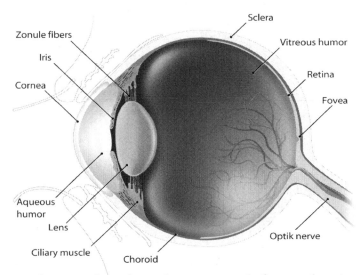

Sclera
Zonule fibers
Vitreous humor
Iris
Retina
Cornea
Fovea
Aqueous humor
Lens
Optik nerve
Ciliary muscle
Choroid

normal aging, but they also can result from other issues such as trauma, sun exposure, or diseases. To understand how any cataract forms, it's helpful to understand the makeup of the lens of your eyeball. The lens is made up mostly of protein and water. The protein is arranged in such a way that when light passes through it to get to the retina, it does so without distortion.

As people age, however, changes in the eye cause protein to break down and clump together, creating a buildup that hardens and blurs your vision. More specifically, the lens thickens, becoming less flexible and transparent. At first, the clouding involves a small area, but over time it increases in size, density, and color, eventually engulfing the entire lens. Your vision is affected because the clumping scatters light coming through the lens in such a way that a sharply defined image can't reach the retina. Your lens no longer has the ability to adjust appropriately to see up close or far away. Instead, everything you see is faded, distorted, or blurred.

How the Eye Works

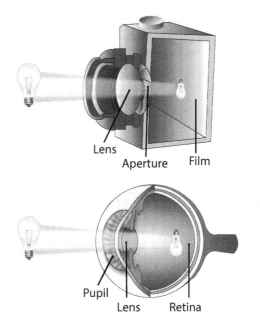

The human eye works much like a camera. In a camera, an image passes through the lens and strikes the film, where it is imprinted into the film. In the eye, an image passes through the lens onto the retina. The image message travels through the optic nerve to the brain, where it is "interpreted."

Types of Cataracts

Eye surgeons have different ways of classifying cataracts based on their location within the lens. The three basic types are *nuclear, cortical,* and *subcapsular,* as explained in the text that follows.

Other types of cataracts, which are not caused by aging, are named according to their underlying origin. For example, these include *congenital* and *traumatic* cataracts.

Nuclear Cataracts

Nuclear cataracts are the most common type of cataract. They form in the center, or *nucleus,* of the eye. They can start forming when you're only in your forties or fifties, but they usually don't significantly affect vision until you're in your sixties and seventies. In fact, by age seventy most men and women have some degree of clouding. Nuclear sclerotic cataracts cause yellow tinting that can eventually harden into a dense yellow or brownish yellow center. Vision gradually deteriorates with symptoms ranging from blurring and seeing halos around objects to having difficulty in distinguishing color or contrasts.

Cortical Cataracts

Cortical cataracts develop along the edge (*cortex*) of the lens. They begin as streaks of whitish, wedge-shaped growths that eventually extend, like the spokes of a wheel, from the edge into the center of the lens. Because of this pattern, light tends to scatter when it hits the lens, causing initial problems with glare. Although older adults can develop cortical cataracts, they're a common problem in diabetics of all ages.

Posterior Subcapsular Cataracts

Posterior subcapsular cataracts form at the back of the lens, directly below the pocket or membrane that surrounds the lens. These cataracts begin as small cloudy areas blocking the path of light to the retina, causing light to scatter rather than remain focused. Symptoms include trouble seeing close-up for reading and sensitivity to bright light, causing severe glare. These cataracts tend to develop relatively quickly, in months rather than years. Although posterior subcapsular cataracts can be related to aging, they're more commonly associated with diabetes and prolonged use of prednisone or other prescription steroids. And, they tend to be seen in younger patients.

Nuclear Cataract

A nuclear cataract is the most common type of cataract. It can cloud the entire lens

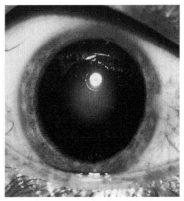

© 2015 American Academy of Ophthalmology

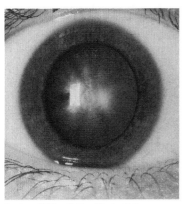

Cortical Cataract

A cortical cataract forms as a wedge on the lens and gradually extends "spokes" toward the center of the lens.

Courtesy of NIH—National Eye Institute

Posterior Subcapsular Cataract

A subcapsular cataract forms toward the back of the lens and interferes with incoming light.

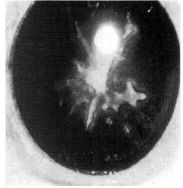

© 2015 American Academy of Ophthalmology

Congenital Cataracts

Unlike cataracts that develop as part of aging, congenital cataracts are present at birth. Although they can be associated with another medical condition, such as Down's syndrome, they also may be caused by genetics or a mother's health during pregnancy. If a woman experiences an infection such as German measles, for instance, her baby may be at risk for congenital cataracts. Cataracts that develop later in childhood are sometimes referred to as *pediatric cataracts*. Although they may be tied to other health conditions, they also can be caused by traumatic injuries to the eye. Damage can take months to years to develop. Congenital and pediatric cataracts are relatively rare. They occur in approximately 3 out of 10,000 children.

Traumatic Cataracts

Traumatic cataracts are cataracts that result from traumas to the eye such as a blunt force, a penetrating injury, or exposure to certain chemicals. They can develop immediately or years later. The cataract forms at the site of the injury, which may involve the entire lens. As noted earlier, traumatic events to the eye are often the source of pediatric cataracts.

Immature and Mature Cataracts

Although most cataracts develop gradually, some individuals may experience rapid growth, particularly if several areas of the lens are affected. In either case, a cataract's natural progression from immature to mature is such that at first the clouding is not visible to the naked eye. You likely won't have noticed it because you aren't having any problems with your vision. The only way your eye doctor knows the cataract is forming is through a comprehensive eye examination.

As time passes, cataracts can advance to a more mature stage when they may be apparent to the naked eye. The cataracts may make the pupil appear milky white or totally opaque. At this stage, the cataract is sometimes referred to as a *mature white cataract.* At one time, ophthalmologists advised patients to delay surgery until the cataract was "ripe," but today they intervene relatively early to preserve a patient's vision.

Mature Brown Cataracts

Mature brown cataracts have progressed to the point of becoming hardened. Eye doctors often see them in older patients who haven't visited an eye doctor in many years. Over time, the protein clumps that form the cataract become very cloudy and are tinged a deep brown, which can affect the ability to distinguish colors. Mature brown cataracts also are often so dense at the center that removing them safely can be challenging. Routine eye examinations can eliminate the development of such advanced cataracts.

Cataract Symptoms

A cataract may cause no visual disturbances at first because the clouding affects only a small part of the lens, but as it grows, scattering even more light trying to reach the retina, a variety of symptoms occur. You may notice:

- painless clouding, blurring, and dimming of vision
- difficulty seeing at night or in reduced light
- sensitivity to light and glare
- presence of "halos" and glare from the sun or oncoming headlights at night
- faded and yellow colors
- need for brighter light for reading and other close-up activities
- frequent changes in either eyeglass or contact lens prescriptions
- double vision within one eye

Although there's no specific order to these early symptoms, eventually they'll interfere with your vision. People often describe the experience as looking through a frosty or fogged-over window. Others say their vision is like viewing the muted images of an impressionist painting. The effects make it difficult to see distant objects, identify facial expressions, and recognize color intensity. The impaired vision also affects one's ability to carry out activities of daily living, including driving. Although cataracts cause visual difficulties, they don't cause discomfort such as itching, burning, or aching, unless they become quite large.

At first, cataract-related symptoms can be treated with stronger lighting and up-to-date eyeglass prescriptions. But eventually, the only way to restore impaired vision is with surgery to remove the cloudy lens and replace it.

How Cataracts Develop

Cataract development or progression varies widely. Your ophthalmologist cannot predict with accuracy when you'll need surgery because cataracts develop at varying rates. In the early stages of a nuclear sclerotic cataract, for instance, the progress can be so slow that you're not even aware that your vision is affected. Sometimes patients become so adept at adapting to their diminished vision that they're surprised after surgery just how well they can see.

In most cases, cataracts don't harm other parts of the eye. (In a small percentage of patients, however, enlarged cataracts can increase the fluid pressure in the eye, causing damage to the optic nerve.) Cataracts also don't "spread" from one eye to the other, even though most people eventually develop them in both eyes. Even though you may get cataracts in both eyes, they don't necessarily occur in the same way in each eye—one cataract develops slower or more quickly than the other one.

Cataract Causes and Risk Factors

As noted earlier, advancing age is the primary risk factor for cataracts. Yet other issues can also increase the likelihood of developing cataracts, even in younger people. Although researchers still don't know why the lens of the eye changes as you get older, they've identified several medical and lifestyle factors that seem to hasten cataract development.

Chronic illnesses

High blood pressure and obesity may increase your risk for cataracts, but diabetes is the most common chronic illness associated with non-age-related or early cataracts. Failing to keep your blood sugar controlled can trigger biochemical changes in the lens that accelerate the formation of a cataract. Diabetic retinopathy, a serious complication, can also impact your cataract and its treatment.

Prolonged corticosteroid or steroid use. Although oral and inhaled prescription steroids are successful treatments for conditions such as asthma, ulcerative colitis, and other chronic conditions, long-term use of these drugs can lead to cataracts sooner rather than later. Other medications such as cholesterol-lowering medications and anti-seizure medications can also be a trigger for long term growth of cataracts. If you've been taking any drug, particularly prednisone or similar steroid medications, you should see your eye doctor regularly.

Eye issues/injuries. Any number of eye problems can increase your risk of developing cataracts. Glaucoma and its treatment, including eye drops and surgery, pose a high risk for cataracts. Penetrating and blunt-force injuries, previous surgeries, and other eye conditions also can cause cataract formation, even years after the event. Furthermore, if you're extremely nearsighted or farsighted, your ophthalmologist will want to monitor you closely because both these vision problems can lead to early cataracts.

Smoking

Studies repeatedly confirm that tobacco plays a prominent role in the development of cataracts. When cigarette smoke enters the body it enhances production of chemical particles called *oxidants* or *oxygen-free radicals,* which damage cells throughout the body, including those in the eye. Overproduction of these microscopic by-products causes lens proteins to clump into a cataract much earlier and quicker in smokers compared to non-smokers. Researchers continue to focus on the major role of oxidants in the development of cataracts.

Genetics

Heredity plays a lesser role in the risk factors for the development of cataracts. Yet certain diseases that run in families can increase a person's susceptibility for cataracts. For example, cataracts are a common complication for those with *retinitis pigmentosa,* a disorder that damages the cells (called *rods*) in the retina that control night vision. Heredity may also be a factor in congenital or pediatric cataracts, which usually involve abnormalities in the shape or structure of the lens and surrounding membrane that lead to the clouding. Scientists are investigating possible causes of both adult and congenital cataracts. As for ethnicity and race, data suggests that some groups, such as African Americans, experience a higher rate of cataracts. But this is likely related to the higher rates of certain diseases, such as diabetes, in these populations, which already creates an increased risk of developing cataracts.

Preventing Cataracts

Because doctors don't have answers to all questions about how cataracts develop, they also don't have specific ways to stop them from forming. There are strategies, however, that may help you prevent or slow the formation of cataracts. You can't reverse the aging process, but you can take practical steps to protect your eyes from cataracts and other eye diseases.

Managing Your Health Issues

If you have a chronic condition that may increase your risk of cataracts, you need to manage it carefully. Researchers know, for instance, that uncontrolled blood glucose or sugar levels connected to diabetes can lead to biochemical changes in the lens that trigger several types of cataracts. Monitoring all of your health issues, particularly a chronic illness, may reduce your risk.

Quit Smoking

Studies have shown that smokers double their risk of developing cataracts over nonsmokers. The more heavily they smoke, the greater the susceptibility. There are many health reasons to quit smoking, and protecting your eyes against early and severe cataracts is an especially important one. Determining which smoking cessation method works best for you—medication, counseling, or classes—can be helpful.

Protect Your Eyes from the Sun

The ultraviolet rays emitted by the sun have destructive properties that can promote cataracts. Penetrating the outer layers of the skin, *ultraviolet-B (UVB),* in particular, is believed to cause changes in the lens that eventually lead to clouding. Deeper *ultraviolet-A (UVA)* rays promote the release of damaging oxygen-free radicals, which also play a role. Wearing sunglasses every time you're outside can be effective in blocking damaging rays.

Eat Healthfully

Scientists have yet to prove conclusively how a diet rich in vitamins and minerals might be linked to avoiding cataracts. But evidence suggests that eating a variety of fruits and vegetables every day provides many of the

11

antioxidants and other nutrients necessary to maintain healthy eyes. One British study, called the *EPIC-Oxford Cohort,* even suggests a significant decrease in cataract risk among some of the 65,000 participants, including 27,640 individuals older than age forty. Of this group, vegetarians, fish eaters, and vegans experienced drops of 30 percent, 21 percent, and 40 percent respectively in their risk for cataracts. Among meat eaters, the more ounces they consumed per day, the higher their cataract risk. Further research is needed on the exact role diet plays in preventing or slowing cataracts. But foods rich in vitamins and minerals likely will help you maintain good eye health.

Schedule Regular Eye Examinations

Comprehensive eye examinations can detect eye diseases, including cataracts, at their earliest stages. Even though age-related cataracts develop over years, undergoing routine exams helps your doctor keep track of their progress so they can be addressed when they start causing vision problems. Your eye care professional will suggest an appropriate schedule for you, which will likely include yearly exams if you are older.

2

Getting a Diagnosis

Because visual loss with cataracts can be slow and progressive, diagnosing them early and having your doctor keep track of them is important. You likely won't need surgery immediately, but you may need adjustments to your eyeglass or contact lens prescription to accommodate your diminished vision. With routine comprehensive eye examinations your eye care professional not only can determine the type and severity of your cataract early, but can also recommend the best treatment plan.

Who Diagnoses Cataracts?

There are several types of eye care professionals who may play a role in diagnosing and treating your cataracts. Although primary care physicians often perform basic or cursory eye exams, especially if they detect a related health issue, only ophthalmologists and optometrists are specially trained to evaluate your vision.

It's important to understand the roles of ophthalmologists and optometrists. They have different training, capabilities, and skills, especially in relation to eye diseases, such as cataracts, that might be causing your diminished vision.

Ophthalmologists

Ophthalmologists are specialty physicians who focus on the diagnosis, treatment, and care of the eyes. As medical doctors, they're not only trained to perform comprehensive eye exams and prescribe glasses, but they also can diagnose and treat eye diseases. General ophthalmologists provide a spectrum of eye care, from routine exams to surgical and other medical treatments. They have the skills and experience not only to remove your cataracts, but also to determine if and when you're ready for surgery.

Some ophthalmologists have chosen to focus on certain eye conditions and have undergone advanced training to do so. Ophthalmologists who are retina specialists or perhaps cornea specialists are examples. Even if an ophthalmologist has a special interest in cataract or other treatment, he or she may still offer comprehensive services.

Whether they eventually become generalists or specialists, ophthalmologists have undergone rigorous training that begins with four years of medical school after college, followed by a one year general medical internship. To be licensed by any state, they also must complete three or more years of residency or hands-on training supervised by experienced ophthalmologists. Cataract care is a core competency in that training. Although many ophthalmologists enter the workforce after graduating from residency, others hone their skills through an additional one- or two-year fellowship. Fellowships give physicians the opportunity to concentrate on a specific area, or *subspecialty,* by working closely for a time with physicians experienced in that field. In ophthalmology, there are many fellowship options, including retinal and corneal surgery, pediatric ophthalmology, and even oculo-plastic surgery.

Optometrists

Optometrists play an important role in providing primary eye care, including diagnosing cataracts and assessing their impact on a person's lifestyle. They also make routine referrals to ophthalmologists, who are qualified to treat cataracts. To be licensed as an optometrist in any state, candidates must complete four years of college and a four-year accredited doctor of optometry program. Some also undergo residency or other training as well as earn American Board of Optometry certification. Board certification recognizes that an optometrist has exceeded the basic requirements of the profession by meeting certain standards. That includes proof of clinical experience and passage of a national exam.

An optometrist's preparation allows him or her to perform complete eye exams, diagnose vision problems, and prescribe eyeglasses, contact lenses, and some medications. Because optometrists don't perform eye surgery, they typically refer cataract patients to an ophthalmologist.

Your Eye Exam

Regular eye exams, especially as you get older, are important not only for adjusting your eyeglasses or contact lenses, but also for diagnosing common eye conditions. These may include cataracts as well as glaucoma—the buildup of excess pressure in the eyeball—and age-related macular degeneration—the deterioration of light-sensitive tissue or macula at the back of the eye.

Because cataracts develop unpredictably over time it's important that your eye doctor routinely evaluate their progression so that you receive timely treatment. The further your cataract has advanced, the greater the risk for surgical complications.

To assess your eye health, your optometrist or ophthalmologist uses a variety of tests and procedures. Their tools range from a simple eye chart to a high-powered microscope for examining the structures inside the eye. Every aspect of your eye health, including your central and peripheral or side vision, is evaluated. For part of the exam, your pupils are dilated or widened with special drops to give the doctor a clear view inside.

Your doctor will begin with your medical history before assessing your vision, measuring your refractive error, examining the exterior and interior of your eyeball, and gauging your eye pressure. Depending on your symptoms, he or she may add additional checks, such as ultrasound or a brightness acuity test (BAT). Together they not only produce a picture of how your eyes are moving and functioning separately and together, but they also yield specific information about any eye issues, especially cataracts.

Medical/Eye Health History

Understanding your general and eye health history is critical in diagnosing and treating cataracts. Although age is certainly a determining factor, so are specific issues such as diabetes, steroid use, cardiac problems, and even previous eye conditions or trauma. Because these conditions can raise the risk for certain types of cataracts or impact your treatment, they're of particular interest.

Medical History

Although your ophthalmologist is assessing the totality of your health, he or she is likely to focus on specific factors that come to light from your medical history and may have a bearing on your cataract.

People with diabetes, for instance, are more likely to develop cataracts of several types and do so at a younger age than other people. As such, your eye doctor will be alert to any signs of diabetic retinopathy because it's not only a complication of diabetes, but also can be a factor in cataract treatment. Retinopathy is caused by damage to the blood vessels in the light-sensitive tissue of the retina.

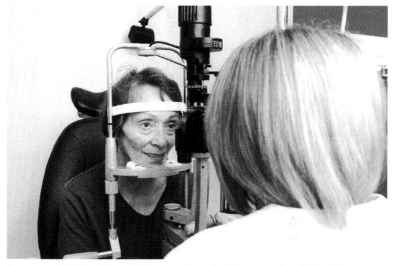

To assess a patient's eyes for cataracts, an ophthalmologist uses a device called a slit lamp to perform a microscopic evaluation of the eye's interior.

Your eye doctor is also concerned about your blood glucose levels—are they within normal range, especially if you're having cataract surgery?

Likewise, because long-term steroid use is linked to increased risk for subcapsular cataracts, cataracts that develop under the lens capsule, you'll likely be asked about your prescriptions. Many people suffering from chronic conditions, ranging from arthritis to ulcerative colitis or inflammation of the bowel, rely on these anti-inflammatory drugs long term for pain relief. Keep in mind, however, that even though prednisone is what most people associate with prescription steroids, there are many other drugs that contain steroidal ingredients. So when your doctor asks, for instance, if you've ever had a knee injection for arthritis or used nose sprays for allergies or inhalers for asthma, he or she is confirming what might be causing your cataract. That information is especially important if you're developing a cataract at a younger age.

Your eye surgeon also wants to know your cardio-vascular or heart risk factors to make sure that if you need surgery, you're medically stable enough to get through it safely. Since high blood pressure is the most common reason to cancel any operation, he or she will check that yours is under control. The presence of any health issue doesn't change the surgical treatment for a cataract, but your doctor will take into account any condition that could delay or impede successful treatment.

Eye Health

Although your general health history is important, your ophthalmologist is specifically concerned about your eye health. Knowing what's occurred to your eye in the past may explain why you're developing a cataract now, especially if it's clearly not age-related. Moreover, understanding what other eye issues you might be experiencing currently is critical in determining how to move forward.

Because cataracts in middle-aged adults are often the result of childhood injury or trauma to the eye, your doctor is likely to ask about such injuries if you're only in your thirties or forties and your lens is clouding. You may not recall being hit in the eye with a baseball bat, for instance, but your doctor will ask about such events because they may explain why a cataract is developing now.

He or she will also be interested if you've had previous surgeries on the eye or if you experienced *amblyopia* or lazy eye as a youngster. Besides being linked to childhood cataracts, lazy eye can cause residual problems in adults. It may explain why vision in an eye that has just developed a cataract is so much worse than the cataract would normally trigger at this point.

Your ophthalmologist will be alert to other eye conditions not only because they're key to your overall vision, but also because they may impact how and when your cataract is treated. If you have age-related macular degeneration, for instance, you have the same risk for developing cataracts as a normal-vision person. Yet the challenge for your eye doctor in terms of your cataract surgery is to determine how much of your vision loss is actually due to each condition. Likewise, even though glaucoma causes vision loss on its own, cataracts can worsen the situation. Conversely, the clouding also can form in response to severe eye pressure buildup.

Whatever your eye health issues, your doctor needs to know about them to make treatment recommendations.

Vision Assessment

Because normal aging and various eye issues, including cataracts, can cause your vision to blur over time, assessing your acuity or sharpness is critical. Your doctor needs to know if and by how much your ability to see well is affected, whether or not a cataract is the source.

Normal vision, which is often referred to as 20/20, means that you can see people or objects clearly at 20 feet. Any variation on that number indicates that you likely need corrective lenses. If your vision in one eye is 20/100, for instance, you see at 20 feet what someone with normal vision sees at 100 feet. Although 20/20 vision is an optimal reading, it doesn't mean that you have perfect sight. It is possible that other problems may be compromising your vision; they may include such things as peripheral or side vision, eye coordination, depth perception, focusing capacity, and color vision.

Although your doctor will assess those skills during other parts of the exam, for visual acuity he or she relies on a test in use since the mid-1800s: The *Snellen* or "big E" block letter chart. You're likely familiar with its role in measuring how well you can see at various distances. Although there are variations, the Snellen chart generally consists of eleven rows of progressively smaller capital letters. Normally you'd stand twenty feet from a paper

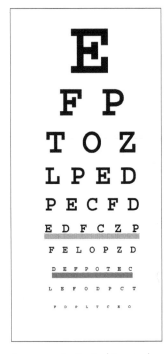

An eye examination to determine how well you see typically includes the use of a Snellen eye chart, which has progressively smaller letters on each line.

Snellen chart, but because most doctors' examining rooms don't have that kind of space, you'll likely be looking at an electronic version calibrated to accommodate for distance.

Because your eyes are not identical (one is usually weaker than the other), each eye is measured independently. During the test, you'll be asked to cover one eye as you indicate what you can or can't read with the other. The smallest line you can see clearly indicates your visual acuity. If you can only decipher the large "E" atop the chart clearly, your vision is 20/200, which indicates poor vision. If you can read the eighth line with no hesitation, however, you have normal 20/20 sight. Deciphering the three smallest lines, particularly the last one, suggests better than normal acuity.

Most doctors also check a patient's vision with their existing eyeglasses to see if changing the prescription will actually improve acuity. Because Medicare or private health insurance wants to know that you have the best vision possible with your current or new correction before paying for cataract surgery, it's important for your doctor to determine how much he or she can improve your vision with eyeglasses first.

Although a vision assessment can indicate the extent to which cataracts might be clouding your sight, it doesn't confirm their actual presence. Your doctor will need to evaluate each eye further to diagnose what's actually occurring, whether it's cataracts or another eye condition.

Determining Refractive Error

Refractive error is a term doctors use to describe the optical imperfections that prevent the eye from properly focusing light. It occurs when light rays don't bend or *refract* correctly in reaching the retina, ultimately resulting in blurry or distorted vision. Determining the type and degree of your refractive error is necessary in prescribing proper eyeglass or contact lens power.

Normally, your eye creates a clear, sharp image because the cornea and lens focus rays of light onto the retina by bending them in a specific way to reach it. But sometimes the natural length of your eye or the curvature of your cornea or lens can get in the way of that process, making it difficult to focus properly. The ability of your eye to focus light sharply on the retina is based primarily on your eyeball's anatomy. You're likely already familiar with the most common refractive errors.

Myopia or Nearsightedness

With myopia, your cornea is curved too steeply or your eyeball is too long relative to the focusing power of the cornea and lens. Light rays from distant objects

Myopia

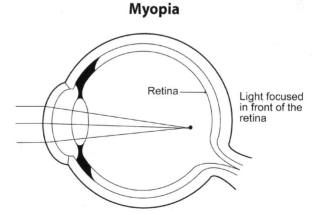

Retina

Light focused in front of the retina

Also referred to as being nearsighted, myopia causes images to focus in front of the retina, allowing you to see images close up better than images in the distance.

21

have to bend severely to reach the retina and instead focus in front of it, blurring distant objects. Myopia causes difficulty seeing far away.

Hyperopia

Hyperopia or farsightedness means your eyeball is too short relative to the combined focusing power of the cornea and lens. That means light rays focus on a point beyond the retina, causing blurring of near objects. Hyperopia causes difficulty in seeing things near.

Hyperopia

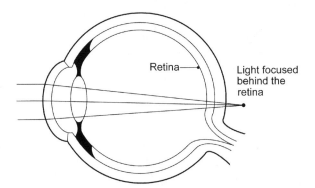

More commonly known as being farsighted, hyperopia causes light rays to focus behind the retina. As a result, you can see objects in the distance more clearly than those up close.

Presbyopia

Presbyopia is the inability of aging eyes to accommodate very close-up vision. With normal vision, you're able to see clearly because the lens is elastic enough to change shape. When necessary, it becomes thicker and more curved to bring light rays reflecting very close objects into sharp focus on the retina. As you age, however, the lens loses that flexibility. It's less able to make this accommodation. Eventually, light no longer can be focused, making it difficult to focus on very, very close or "arm's-length" ranges.

Presbyopia

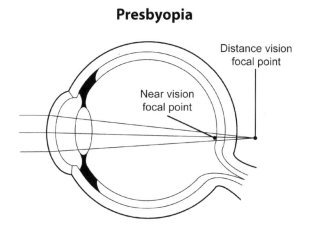

Presbyopia makes ability difficult to see objects that are very close. This is a result of the lens losing its elasticity and ability to change shape to bring close-up objects into focus.

Astigmatism or Blurriness Due to the Irregular Shaped Cornea

Under normal circumstances, light rays entering the eye are bent into a singular focal point on the retina at the back of the eye to achieve sharp vision. But with astigmatism the cornea is unevenly curved. It looks much like a football rather than naturally spherical or round.

Astigmatism

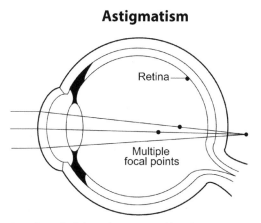

With astigmatism, objects both far and near appear blurry because the curvature of the cornea prevents light rays from uniformly focusing on the retina.

This irregular curvature prevents light from properly hitting the retina. Instead, it refracts onto different parts of the cornea in differing degrees. Because the rays are dispersed everywhere, the lens can't bring them into single retinal focus. Instead, objects appear distorted. Because astigmatism frequently occurs with nearsightedness and farsightedness, it can blur your vision at any distance. It can also compound other blurriness.

Refractive Error Testing

Refraction error testing is part of every comprehensive eye examine. Your doctor needs to determine how much power is necessary to enable you to have normal, focused vision. He or she relies on manual and/or automated instruments to detect the type and degree of your refractive error. This evaluation usually involves two parts: the objective portion during which you don't provide feedback, and the subjective portion when you'll be asked to respond.

To obtain an objective refractive reading, ophthalmologists use an instrument called a *retinoscope*. It's a handheld device that helps determine if and to what degree you're having difficulty seeing up close or far away. With no input from you, the doctor shines a light through the pupil by moving the retinoscope back and forth in front of each eye. How the retina reflects or responds to those movements determines your level of nearsightedness, farsightedness, or another refractive error. By shining the light additionally through a series of lenses flashed in front of the eye, he or she also can narrow your prescription.

Retinoscopy is considered extremely accurate. Yet your doctor will likely combine it with results from a *phoropter* test that involves your feedback. The phoropter is an imposing, albeit efficient, instrument for subjectively determining an individual's refractive error and correction. Placed in front of your face, it looks like a pair of jumbo-sized glasses with attached lenses and dials that your doctor manipulates. As you're seated, you'll be asked to look through the machine's eyepieces to an "E" chart. Your eye professional obtains the correct refractive measurement by guiding you through multiple lens changes. As you read the letters on the eye chart, the doctor or technician will ask, "Which is better, one or two?", referring to which lens enables you to see the chart with greater clarity.

Refractive errors are corrected by altering the angle of rays before they reach the surface of the cornea so the lens of the eye can focus them correctly on the retina. That's achieved through eyeglasses, contact lenses, or refractive surgery, such as LASIK (*laser in situ keratomileusis*).

Your doctor needs to know the extent of your diminished eyesight not only to ensure that your eyeglass prescription gives you the best possible vision, but also because it may have a bearing on the artificial lens your doctor inserts during cataract surgery. Medicare and other insurers don't pay to surgically correct refractive errors, such as farsightedness, nearsightedness, astigmatism, or presbyopia.

Examining the Eyeball

Your eye care professional can learn much about the health and function of your eyes by examining both the outside and inside of your eyeball. Every comprehensive eye exam includes simple tracking tests to make sure that your eyes move normally together and that your pupils are responding correctly to light. It also involves a thorough evaluation of your eyeball structures. Even though a cataract forms on the lens, it's critical for your eye doctor to know the status of each component contributing to your vision. He or she begins by making sure that every external feature is healthy, from the *sclera,* or white area, surrounding your iris and pupils to your eyelids.

Your eyelids are of particular concern because they can put your recovery after cataract surgery at risk. For instance, an untreated infection, called *blepharitis,* can lead to a more serious, albeit rare, condition called *endophthalmitis,* which could cost you your vision. It's an inflammation of the inside of the eye associated with any eye surgery. Even though it's rare, it's the reason you'll want to carefully follow your doctor's instructions regarding eye care and antibiotics after your procedure. Likewise, if your lower eyelid folds in or out abnormally you may be at risk for corneal problems that also can cause serious infection and potential visual loss.

Your doctor can identify problems with your eyelid during a visual inspection. But he or she also will rely on a diagnostic gold standard to investigate further. The slit lamp, or biomicroscope, combines a high-powered "slit" or intense line of light with a microscope to illuminate and magnify structures at the front and back of the eye. It not only allows your doctor to evaluate the health of every part of your eye, but also to diagnose issues such as cataracts.

To perform the test, you'll be asked to place your chin on the lamp's chin rest as your doctor shines the slit light on the frontal structures of your eyes to illuminate them. He or she will look through a set of *oculars,* eyepieces similar to those you'd find on any science lab microscope, to examine the cornea, iris, and lens. The microscope allows for close evaluation of those and other structures, such as the *vitreous gel,* the thick gel that fills the middle of the eyeball.

Viewing the Interior Eye with Dilation

Although the slit lamp shines a light on the frontal structures of your eye, dilating, or enlarging the pupils is important because it allows for a full evaluation of the interior of your eye, especially the back area, where the retina, macula, and optic nerve are located.

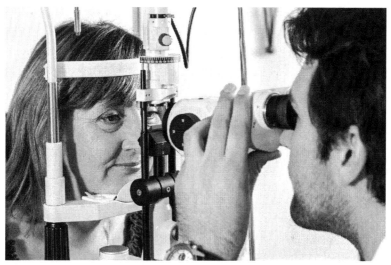

An ophthalmologist uses eye drops to dilate your pupils. By enlarging the pupils, the doctor is able to better see the structures inside the eye.

To help the light reach the deepest structures, your doctor applies special medicated drops that either stimulate the muscles that cause your pupil to widen or relax the muscles that cause them to restrict. Sometimes doctors do both. By changing the width and height of the light beam and placing additional magnifying lenses (referred to as *indirect ophthalmoscopy*) in front of your eyes, your doctor can get a wider view of the retina or back of the eye.

In terms of cataracts, the slit lamp provides useful information after your eyes are dilated. Because the lamp produces a three-dimensional view (top, middle, and bottom) of your clouded lens, your doctor is able to classify and grade the cataract with accuracy. He or she not only can determine its size and progression, but also identify multiple types if you have more than one cataract, which can occur.

Although the slit lamp is valuable in diagnosing cataracts, your eye surgeon also may use it in fine-tuning his or her surgical treatment plan. Since the microscope in the operating room doesn't produce the same detailed view of your cataract as the slit lamp, your doctor may rely on this examination to identify other factors, such as previous eye trauma or issues with the cornea, lens, or pupil, which could make cataract surgery more difficult later.

Whatever the results, the slit lamp evaluation is effective and painless, even though having your pupils dilated may be slightly inconvenient. You'll likely have difficulty focusing for several hours so you'll want to have someone drive you home after the appointment. Also, because you'll be more sensitive to sunlight than usual, you'll want to wear sunglasses for a few hours after the evaluation.

Measuring Eye Pressure

Measuring the pressure inside of your eyes, referred to as *intraocular pressure (IOP),* is an important part of any comprehensive eye exam. Your physician wants to ensure that you're not at risk for or already have *glaucoma,* a condition that causes damage to the optic nerve. It's caused by a buildup of pressure because the fluid, called *aqueous humor,* can't drain properly. Glaucoma not only diminishes sight, but also can affect cataracts *and* may be affected by them.

Testing Pressure

Intraocular pressure is gauged in *millimeters (mm) of mercury (Hg),* the same measurement unit used for blood pressure. Normal intraocular pressure ranges from 10 to 21 mm/Hg, with the average between 14 and 16 mm/Hg. Greater than 22 mm/Hg generally means you're at risk for glaucoma. The *tonometry* tests to gauge and track eye pressures are both simple and painless. The most common is the air puff test, technically referred to as *noncontact tonometry* or *NCT.* The gold standard, however, is *Goldmann applanation tonometry,* a test based on an

Glaucoma

Part of your eye exam will test the internal pressure of your eye. Too much pressure can cause glaucoma, a condition caused by the buildup of too much fluid in the eyeball. If left untreated, glaucoma can damage the optic nerve.

instrument developed by Swiss ophthalmologist Hans Goldmann.

To conduct the air puff test, you'll be asked to place your chin on the brace of the tonometer and concentrate on a light emitting from inside. The machine then points a small jet directly at your eye, delivering a quick puff of air onto the surface to flatten the cornea. It calculates the pressure by measuring the eye's resistance to the puff. Because the tonometer never touches your eye, there's no discomfort in the split second the test takes.

Although the air puff test is a widespread screening tool for glaucoma, many eye professionals believe that applanation tonometry yields a much more accurate assessment of intraocular pressure. It's considered a better tool for two reasons. First, the tip of the probe actually makes contact with the eye for several seconds. Second, because the doctor is viewing the eye through the microscopic lens of a slit lamp while measuring the pressure, he or she can fine-tune the measurement.

For applanation tonometry, the doctor applies numbing drops infused with yellow *fluorescein* dye to the eyes. Because it glows under the tonometer's cobalt blue light, the dye will allow a much better view inside the eye. You're asked to rest your chin on the brace of a slit lamp, where the applanation tonometer is mounted. Your doctor presses the tip of a small probe on the surface of the eye to make an indentation on the cornea. Again, the pressure is measured by how much force is needed to flatten the cornea.

Because there are typically no early warning signs for glaucoma, monitoring your vision regularly, especially as you age, is critical. In terms of cataracts, however, there are other reasons your doctor wants to know if you have glaucoma. Because each condition can affect the other, he or she needs to know the extent of both to make the best treatment recommendations.

Other Tests

Your eye doctor has other tests that he or she can use to learn more about a cataract and/or how it might be affecting your day-to-day living. Ultrasound and laser technologies, for instance, are sometimes employed to further measure the lens and document the areas and severity of the clouding. Specialized testing isn't usually included in a routine comprehensive eye exam. Instead, your ophthalmologist likely will order it as a follow-up. It may also be part of an evaluation if you've been referred for treatment to a cataract surgeon. For instance, if your eye doctor suspects your cataract is causing undue glare, he or she may order an additional check.

Brightness Acuity Testing (BAT)

Brightness acuity testing (BAT) helps your eye doctor determine how bright light is affecting your vision. It can also be an indicator as to whether or not your cataract is causing you problems in completing your day-to-day tasks.

Because a common symptom of any lens clouding is diminished vision in the glare of bright lights, physicians often use this test to measure a patient's visual acuity by simulating such conditions. They may order it if the questionnaire you complete about your lifestyle and daily activities suggests that you have difficulty with certain types of bright indoor or outdoor light.

To conduct brightness acuity testing, your doctor shines a handheld device into your eyes as you're deciphering letters on the eye chart. Vision is measured using light settings that replicate various conditions. The low setting, for instance, is similar to workplace lighting while the high setting mimics oncoming headlights or bright sun. If your visual acuity gets worse during the test, you likely have what's called a "glare disability" brought on by your cataract.

Performing a glare test is particularly useful if there's a difference between your visual acuity in the dim light of the exam room and what you're really experiencing elsewhere. For example, you may have 20/30 vision, but the fact that blinding headlights make you reluctant to drive at night suggests that your cataract needs to be addressed because it's preventing you from doing the things you enjoy.

With the brightness acuity test, your eye doctor can replicate the glare to see if there's a drop in that eye's vision. If it plummets to 20/400, for instance, the test confirms that your cataract is indeed causing a problem with bright light. This information is important to both of you. A cataract that interferes with your ability to carry on normal activities is often a signal that it's time for cataract surgery. The glare test gives your ophthalmologist a measurable way to show Medicare or other insurers that surgery is warranted.

3

Your Intraocular Lens

An *intraocular lens* is an artificial lens that an oph-thalmologist implants in your eye after removing a cataract. Without it, your vision would be severely diminished after cataract removal surgery. With an intraocular lens, however, you'll likely be able to see just as you did with your natural lens, perhaps even better. Today's high-tech intraocular lenses (IOLs) provide a range of optical powers and technical features that restore distance, intermediate, and near vision after cataract surgery.

Development of the Intraocular Lens

The artificial intraocular lens your eye surgeon recommends today was made possible because of the foresight of a British ophthalmologist, Harold Ridley, M.D., more than sixty years ago. He invented the intraocular lens based on a discovery made while treating wounded Royal Air Force fighter pilots for eye injuries during World War II. Dr. Ridley noticed that his patients didn't reject the splinters of *Plexiglas* or *acrylic plastic* from cockpit canopies that had lodged in their eyes during combat missions. Instead, the splinters seemed to float inside the eyeball, unlike glass shards.

That discovery eventually led Dr. Ridley to the implanting of artificial lenses in cataract patients. He sought out an English manufacturer to create the first intraocu-

Intraocular Lens

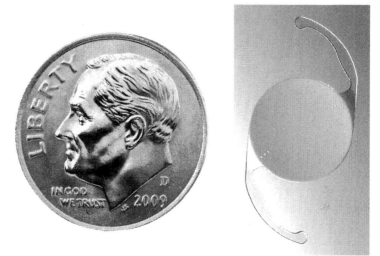

The typical intraocular lens is about two-thirds the size of dime. *Courtesy of Alcon Laboratories, Inc.*

lar lens comprised of plastic materials, similar to those he had observed in the eyes of his fighter pilot patients. Dr. Ridley achieved his first implant in 1949, followed in 1950 by the first permanent implant. In 1952, physicians at Philadelphia's Wills Eye Hospital performed the first intraocular lens surgery in the United States.

Improving the Intraocular Lens

After his initial success, Dr. Ridley continued perfecting the lens and fine-tuning the surgical techniques for implanting it, even in the face of strong opposition from the medical community. Ophthalmologists initially discounted him for even thinking of inserting a foreign object in the eye. In time, however, they accepted the intraocular lens as an effective solution for restoring vision in cataract patients. Some doctors even contributed their own refinements, helping the lens and surgical approach achieve worldwide acceptance.

Other doctors, including several prominent Americans, contributed their own refinements, making it possible for the lens and this surgical approach to achieve worldwide acceptance in the late 1970s.

A decade later, in addition to pioneering what would become the preferred small-incision approach, researchers designed pliable silicone lenses that could be maneuvered safely through tiny incisions. The beauty of the *foldable* intraocular lens, about two-thirds the size of a dime, is that it can be folded and then inserted into the eye; after it's inserted, the lens then expands to its full size. What's more, it can fit into the *posterior,* or back, of the lens capsule, a much more favorable position than the *anterior,* or front, placement that some European doctors used.

Although the Food and Drug Administration (FDA) approved intraocular lenses in 1981 for widespread use, they've undergone continual improvements in design, function, and variety. The lenses your ophthalmologist recommends today have an excellent track record for both safety and effectiveness. They're still soft, pliable, and foldable, making them easier to insert during surgery than any hard lens. The smaller incision reduces the possibility of astigmatism and speeds recovery.

Some types of intraocular lenses can do more than restore only basic far or near vision after a cataract is removed. They can provide distance, intermediate, and near vision, so you may no longer be dependent on eyeglasses. With *premium* lenses, for instance, you may not have to wear bifocals or reading glasses again . However, you'll need to pay out-of-pocket costs for features not considered medically necessary by Medicare or private insurance.

Types of Intraocular Lenses

An important part of your discussion with your eye doctor prior to cataract surgery will be about the type of intraocular lens to be implanted when your natural lens (with the cataract) is removed. The type of IOL you choose will affect how well you see with the naked eye after surgery.

In suggesting an appropriate IOL, your ophthalmologist will want to know what your vision goal is after surgery. Do you want to be free of eyeglasses? Or, do you just mind wearing eyeglasses for certain tasks? In order to get a sense of your day-to-day routine, work responsibilities, and hobbies, your doctor may ask you to complete a questionnaire to get answers to these questions about your lifestyle. For example, knowing that you work at a computer much of the day helps your ophthalmologist determine your best options for lens replacement. He or she will recommend an IOL based on your budget and your priorities. There are three categories of IOLs—single (or mono) focal, multifocal, and accommodating.

Monofocal Intraocular Lenses

Monofocal lenses are the standard lenses that eye surgeons have been implanting in their cataract patients for several decades. They're referred to as *mono* because they provide a singular focus when you're not wearing eyeglasses. Depending on the lens power you and your doctor choose, your eye may see best at far, intermediate, or near distances. Many cataract patients choose a monofocal lens for distant or far vision because it tends to produce very crisp results. If this is your choice, you'll still need eyeglasses for close-up vision, and you may need glasses at all times, depending on your generic, pre-existing astigmatism.

Multifocal Intraocular Lenses

A newer generation of intraocular lenses, multifocal lenses work much like progressive eyeglass lenses in that they provide a visual range in helping patients achieve far, intermediate, and near vision. The surface of the lens is divided into zones of varying optical power to sharpen vision at various distances. As incoming light passes through each zone, it refracts or bends the light, bringing objects or other images into focus. Once the brain learns to select the appropriate zone, the image comes clearly into view. Although visual acuity with multifocal lenses varies from individual to individual, statistics suggest that the majority of people—about 85 percent—no longer need eyeglasses or contact lenses. Those individuals who require eyeglasses, especially for reading and close-up tasks, still experience a marked reduction in their dependence on them.

Multifocal lenses are often referred to as *presbyopia-correcting* lenses because they can restore the close-up vision you lose with age. You may recall, presbyopia is caused by the loss of elasticity in the lens of your eye, making it harder to read or see objects close to you.

Toric Intraocular Lenses

Toric intraocular lenses are a type of monofocal lenses that have a built-in astigmatism correction much like the one you'd achieve with eyeglasses. As you will recall, astigmatism is a defect in the shape or curvature of the cornea that causes distorted or blurred vision. Your doctor may recommend a monofocal intraocular lens with an accompanying eyeglass prescription for the astigmatism or the toric intraocular lens. (Vision-correction surgery for astigmatism is another option you may wish to discuss with your ophthalmologist.)

The toric IOL corrects vision by redirecting light to one focal point on the retina, usually for clear distance vision. Most individuals still need eyeglasses or contact lenses to see images in both near and intermediate vision fields. But, with a toric IOL, you can experience significant improvement in your astigmatism.

Accommodating Intraocular Lenses

Accommodating intraocular lenses are some of the newest advanced features lenses available today. They're designed to help people experience a full range of vision by correcting for presbyopia and astigmatism along with other refractive errors.

Accommodating lenses work by re-creating the natural focusing power of a healthy, young lens. By the time people reach forty, they've usually lost the lens flexibility to focus on close tasks and move from those tasks through other visual ranges with clarity. An accommodating lens attempts to restore that capability by

Toric IOL

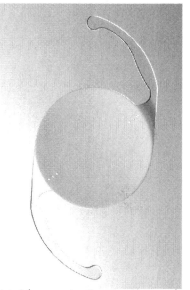

This toric lens corrects astigmatism. Many people choose a toric lens that provides clear distance vision; they wear eyeglasses for near vision. *Courtesy of Alcon Laboratories, Inc.*

flexing in response to normal eye muscle contractions. It differs from a multifocal IOL in that it actually moves backwards and forwards as the eye muscles move, redirecting light onto the retina to bring far, intermediate, and near objects into clear focus. With an accommodating lens, your eye surgeon can't guarantee 20/20 vision and you may even need eyeglasses for some very fine tasks. But, you'll likely experience visual improvement in all ranges. The improvement in vision depends on the strength of your eye's accommodating muscles, which will have been weakened by years of wearing reading glasses; however, after cataract surgery, these muscles can be exercised and strengthened.

Aspheric IOL

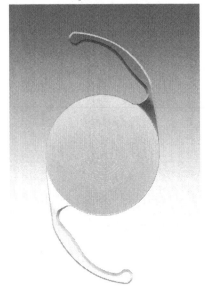

The newer aspherical intraocular lens is flat around the edges. This lens improves vision by making objects appear sharper. The aspheric lens can also improve vision in various lighting conditions. *Courtesy of Alcon Laboratories, Inc.*

Using Two Monofocal Lenses for Monovision

If you need cataract surgery in both eyes, your surgeon may suggest *blended* or *monovision* to accommodate both near and distance vision. With this approach, the surgeon implants a monofocal lens for near or intermediate vision in one eye and a monofocal lens for distance vision in the other eye. Success relies on the brain's ability to adapt, which happens easily for many individuals. People who get the most from monovision frequently have already experienced the same effect with contact lenses for dealing with presbyopia. However, monovision doesn't work well for everyone. If you can't adjust, both your near and far vision may become blurry. You also may experience a loss of depth perception because your eyes aren't working together as they did previously. If your brain can learn to use both lenses, however, a wide range of vision is possible. (Of course, astigmatism must be addressed surgically.)

How Is an Intraocular Lens Made?

As mentioned, most intraocular lenses are slightly more than two-thirds the size of a dime, and they are made of pliable acrylic or silicone plastics that can be folded and inserted through a very small incision. Silicone intraocular lenses were the first foldable models to replace the original rigid lenses. Acrylic lenses are used more often today, even though both materials are biocompatible, meaning they are not harmful to living tissue.

Traditional intraocular lenses are spherically shaped like the eye, meaning the front surface is uniformly curved. However, newer high-tech *aspherical-shaped* multifocal and monofocal lenses are flat around the edges. The design improves image vibrancy, in part by increasing the contrast between color images and their backgrounds. Driving simulator studies have even documented that people wearing aspherical lenses were quicker to put on the simulated brakes after seeing a child chasing a ball into the street than people with spherical lenses.

In addition to providing greater visual clarity, one of the advantages of today's IOLs is that eye surgeons can use a smaller incision to remove the cataract and insert the lens. A smaller incision means improved safety and better results with faster healing.

Placement of the Intraocular Lens

Your doctor will likely place your IOL in the same pocket or bag that held your natural lens before it developed a cataract. This pocket, known as the *posterior capsule,* is a small space directly behind the iris, the colored part of your eye. Doctors prefer this location because it offers many surgical and other advantages to the *anterior,* or front, portion of the pupil where lenses were once routinely implanted, mainly in Europe.

Anterior Lens and Positioning

The anterior positioning of an intraocular lens refers to placing the lens in the anterior, or front, chamber of the eye, a space bounded by the cornea and iris. In the past, anterior intraocular lenses were a standard option for replacing a natural lens after removing a cataract. But to place the rigid plastic lens, ophthalmologists had to make a relatively large (between six- and ten-millimeters)

Placement of IOLs

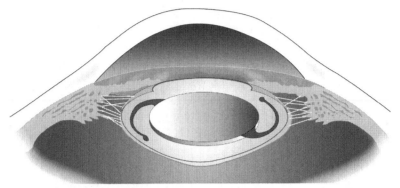

An intraocular lens is inserted in the same capsule (membrane) that held the natural lens. The struts, called *haptics,* on the sides of the lens help hold it in place.

incision through the pupil to access the anterior chamber. The combination of the bulky lens, large incision, and frontal positioning often produced disappointing results, however. Even though anterior lenses have been modified over the years, eye surgeons today usually use them only when the posterior capsule cannot support an implant.

Posterior Lens and Positioning

The posterior positioning of an intraocular lens refers to placing the lens in its natural capsule in back of the pupil and iris. Because a posterior IOL is foldable, an eye surgeon can make a much smaller incision (less than three millimeters) in the cornea of the eye to remove the cataract and then insert the lens, which then expands in the posterior capsule. The natural environment of the pocket offers many advantages. It gives the IOL stability while reducing the potential for visual complications and side effects. Furthermore, because posterior intraocular lenses are made of well-tolerated acrylic or silicone, your eye should accept your implant for a very long time. Once the lens is in place, you shouldn't feel discomfort, other than perhaps the initial healing from your incision.

Your intraocular lens will mimic the natural lens you had before your cataract, only it works better in many cases due to different power and designs.

Common Questions about Intraocular Lenses

Who Manufactures Intraocular Lenses?

Intraocular lenses are manufactured by leading optical device companies. In the United States, companies such as Abbott Medical Optics, Alcon, and Bausch & Lomb are responsible for some of the most reliable and innovative lenses available today. They offer many options in terms of types, optical powers, and other technical features.

How Long Will the Intraocular Lens Last?

No matter which type of intraocular lens you and your eye surgeon choose, it should be permanent. Today's lenses are well tolerated and rarely need to be replaced. Short of major trauma to the eye that might dislocate the lens, the only reason your eye surgeon might suggest removing the lens is if both of you decide that the power isn't correct. Even though your doctor does extensive testing on both you and the lens prior to surgery to determine the best match, 1 in 500 implants is incorrect. If that happens to you, your doctor may replace the original intraocular lens.

Are There Other Options to Lens Removal?

If your ophthalmologist implants an intraocular lens that isn't the right power for you, he or she may suggest a less invasive procedure to replacing the lens. *Piggybacking* involves positioning a second thinner lens atop the first one to strengthen the original focusing power, which is referred to as *diopter*. If your eye surgeon, for instance, implanted a 20-diopter intraocular lens during your cataract surgery, but decided later that you really need a 22-diopter lens, he or she can replace the first lens entirely or else may just piggyback an additional lens onto the first one to achieve the corrected power. In determining what's best for you, your doctor will take various factors into consideration, including the challenges of the first surgery.

Does an Intraocular Lens Protect against Sun Damage to the Eye?

Today's intraocular lenses are designed to protect against light rays that can harm your vision. Although sunlight can cause your eyes to be sensitive, it's the *ultraviolet light rays* emitted by the sun that can damage your sight. Ultraviolet light rays are suspected of causing cataracts and injuring the retina. *High-energy blue light energy rays* also can harm your vision. The sun and other energy sources such as fluorescent or artificial lighting and even computer screens emit these rays. High-energy blue light is considered damaging to the retina. It also may be a risk factor for age-related macular degeneration, which causes central vision loss.

In removing your natural lens, your eye loses its ability to filter some of those harmful rays. Most of today's intraocular lenses, however, are coated with ultraviolet blockers that protect against the sun. Some manufacturers also make intraocular lenses that contain a blue light filter as well.

Even with built-in ultraviolet and blue light blockers, you still need to wear sunglasses. They protect the eyelids from skin cancer and the sclera, or whites, of the eyeball from benign growths that can eventually damage the cornea. Sunglasses also may help prevent or slow the progression of macular degeneration. Besides defending against eye problems, however, they also replace the sun-blocking effects you once had from your cataract. Without the lens clouding, you'll likely be more sensitive to light than in the recent past. Sunglasses will make you more comfortable outdoors.

Does Insurance Pay for an Intraocular Lens?

It's important to remember that Medicare, Medicaid, and private health insurance do not cover every type of intraocular lens. Insurance companies generally reimburse for standard cataract surgery and the insertion of a traditional monofocal lens for distance or near vision correction. But they typically don't reimburse for IOL features that aren't considered medically necessary. They don't cover treatment of vision problems after cataract surgery that can be managed with eyeglasses or contact lenses. That means insurance companies won't pay for premium lenses—multifocal or toric lenses—to specifically address presbyopia or astigmatism.

If you choose a premium lens, you'll likely incur out-of-pocket costs (up to $3,000 per eye) for both the lens and the additional procedures to ensure that the lens is a correct fit. Medicare and private health insurance will still cover the removal of your cataract, including charges for the surgical facility and anesthesiology plus the surgeon's fees, but you'll be responsible for any "extras" related to a premium lens, and/or laser astigmatism correction.

It's important to understand what your eye doctor can provide under Medicare or your private insurance so you won't be disappointed with the results. However, that doesn't mean that you can't achieve a good result. For example, perhaps you've decided that you're comfortable wearing eyeglasses after cataract surgery—you'll still have improved vision.

Many people, however, are willing to pay extra for a premium intraocular lens. They understand that they may still need reading glasses or even over-the-counter "readers" for some close-up tasks, such as reading fine print. But the opportunity to be less dependent on or even "eyeglass-free" with a premium intraocular lens is often worth the additional out-of-pocket costs.

4

Planning for Cataract Surgery

If you're a candidate for cataract surgery, you want to do everything possible to make sure it's safe and successful. There are many things you can learn about the procedure that may help you in planning and making good decisions. Whether you're still looking for an eye surgeon or just want to know how he or she will fit your new intraocular lens, this chapter is intended to help you achieve a successful outcome.

When Should Cataracts Be Removed?

Because cataracts grow slowly, your vision may not be affected for many years. Once the clouding interferes with your work or other normal daily activities, however, your surgeon may recommend surgery. If, for instance, you cannot pass the vision test for your driver's license or you notice that your vision is diminishing, you may be ready for cataract surgery. Your doctor will monitor your cataract's development during routine eye examinations. Cataracts affect vision only by clouding the eye's lens— they do not harm the rest of the eyeball. They should be removed, however, before they become so hardened that they complicate the surgery.

Who Performs Cataract Surgery?

General ophthalmologists perform cataract surgery. You want an ophthalmologist who is experienced in performing cataract surgery and who is also familiar with the latest medical advances and surgical techniques. You can find a qualified cataract surgeon in one of several ways. First, your primary care physician or optometrist will be able to refer you to an ophthalmologist with whom he or she is familiar. Also, if your doctor believes you need a specialist who focuses solely on cataract surgery, you'll likely get a recommendation for such a surgeon.

Board Certification for Ophthalmologists

You also can find names of board-certified eye surgeons through two professional panels—the American Board of Ophthalmology (ABO) and the American Board of Eye Surgery (ABES).

The American Board of Ophthalmology (ABO) was established in 1916 to promote competency and excellence in the field of ophthalmology. The organization certifies ophthalmologists based on their experience and knowledge as demonstrated by rigorous written and oral exams. Becoming an ABO "diplomate" indicates that an ophthalmologist has undergone an eighteen-to-twenty-four-month process to show that he or she is not only competent in treating the human eye, but also committed to continuing education in the profession. You can find an ABO-certified ophthalmologist by visiting www. abop.org. Some ophthalmologists seek additional certification from the American Board of Eye Surgery (ABES). The board was formed in 1985 out of concern that not every eye doctor was adept at the newer technology and surgical techniques that had begun dramatically changing cataract surgery as well as other refractive procedures.

Even though such techniques are virtually universal today, ABES still utilizes a peer-review process to recognize eye surgeons skilled in performing cataract surgery. To be ABES-certified, ophthalmologists must have already completed a minimum of fifty cataract operations that require intraocular lens implantation; they must also have performed a series of surgical procedures with an on-site reviewer observing them. The physician seeking certification must also allow the reviewer access to his or her surgical files to evaluate the outcomes of selected cases. To find an ABES-certified surgeon, contact www.abes.org. Whatever your ophthalmologist's credentials, make sure that he or she has enough experience in performing cataract surgery to minimize the chance of any complications. Because there are risks with every operation, it's important that your eye surgeon is prepared to manage any complication that might develop. Today's cataract surgeries are among the most successful and well tolerated of all medical procedures. Still, you want to make sure that your ophthalmologist is competent and up to date on new technologies.

Measuring Your Eye for an Intraocular Lens

An important part of cataract surgery is finding an intraocular lens that gives you the best possible vision. Your doctor will perform different measurements of your eye to determine your precise intraocular lens power. Fortunately, with the development of sophisticated computerized measuring instruments, your surgeon can accurately calculate the appropriate lens power. Today's computer programs use sophisticated mathematical equations to translate measurements into an IOL power. Being as precise as possible is important because any errors in the dimensions will result in an error in your new lens power. Your doctor will likely use several devices prior to and during surgery to ensure the right intraocular lens fit.

Corneal Curvature

Measuring the shape and curvature of the cornea, the transparent covering on the surface of your eye, is important for selecting an appropriate intraocular lens power. It's also critical in diagnosing the presence and degree of astigmatism, which further impacts the lens choice.

Your doctor will likely use multiple computerized devices to accurately measure your corneal curvature. A medical instrument called a *keratometer*, for instance, uses optical sensors to calculate the horizontal and vertical curvatures of the front surface of your eye based on the shallowest and steepest curves.

Corneal Topography

Another assessment tool, referred to as *corneal topography*, provides even more precise measurements by evaluating thousands of specific points across the entire surface of the cornea and then calculating measurements based on them. The results provide a multidimensional map of your cornea's topography or surface that helps in fitting an intraocular lens.

Although keratometry and corneal topography are standard methods of identifying corneal shape, your surgeon will likely check the results against other computerized instruments. One such system, for instance, enables your surgeon to document the shape, thickness, and structural integrity of your cornea from a picture produced as you stare at a shiny green light.

Cornea-to-Retina Distance

The distance between your cornea and retina (called the *axial length*) is also an important factor in determining the power of your new intraocular lens. In the past, ophthalmologists relied on ultrasound to measure the axial distance; it calculates a measurement based on the echoes made by sound waves as they penetrate the eye and bounce off of its structures.

Corneal Topography

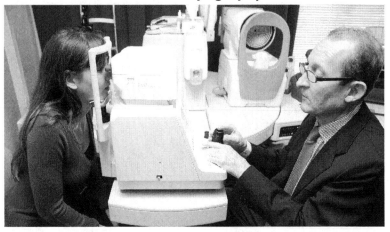

Corneal topography is used to map the surface of the cornea. Prior to cataract surgery, it helps ophthalmologists determine the extent of vision problems caused by the shape of the cornea.

But today there are other sophisticated optical systems that allow eye surgeons to gauge the time required for a beam of infrared light shining through the lens to travel to the retina. In one scan, your doctor can gather several measurements, including the axial length, lens thickness, and depth of the eye's front chamber, all of which are helpful in implanting the right intraocular lens.

Intraoperative Abberometry

Until the advent of innovative technology, called *intraoperative abberometry,* eye surgeons couldn't assess the quality of a cataract patient's vision until weeks after the lens was implanted. Today, however, intraoperative abberometry gives doctors an immediate indication of the best intraocular lens power to insert. This is important because eye surgeons sometimes find an unexpected or unplanned refractive error after removing the cataract, which then changes the IOL power needed.

To perform the analysis, your doctor uses a device attached to the surgical microscope. It scans the eye quickly, providing an unprecedented level of information. The technology can pick up nuances that other measuring devices miss, especially in cases of extreme near- and farsightedness or prior refractive surgery. Based on the results, your surgeon knows how to change or adjust an intraocular lens to fit your needs. Without inserting the lens, your doctor can do a virtual "test drive" to make sure that he or she has chosen the best power for your IOL *before* you leave the operating room.

Intraoperative abberometry reduces the margin of error in selecting an appropriate premium intraocular lens. It also provides the most customized vision correction available today.

Commonly Asked Questions

For most people, the thought of having any surgery creates anxiety. Cataract surgery, in particular, raises a number of concerns because it deals with the eyes. The following questions are those most-often asked by patients considering cataract surgery:

Can I Avoid Surgery with a New Eyeglass Prescription?

As mentioned earlier, just because your vision changes doesn't mean you need cataract surgery immediately. Even if your ophthalmologist suggests surgery, you may wish to ask about other options. Depending on the amount of visual change you have noticed, you may only need a correction in your eyeglass or contacts prescription right now. Because Medicare and other insurers want physicians to at least attempt to improve a cataract patient's vision with better eyeglasses before surgery, ask your ophthalmologist about changing your prescription first.

How Do other Eye and Health Issues Affect the Timing of Cataract Surgery?

Your doctor must take all of your health issues into consideration before surgery. Conditions such as diabetic retinopathy, glaucoma, macular degeneration, high blood pressure, previous infections, and breathing issues can have an impact on your cataract surgery and recovery. Your surgeon will likely confer with your primary care physician and eye specialists you've seen to make sure any medical problems have been addressed and are under control.

What Kind of Restrictions Will I Have after Cataract Surgery? Will I Need Eyeglasses?

With today's cataract surgical techniques, patients no longer have to remain immobile while healing. Recovery is usually short. Other than keeping your micro-incision clean, you'll be back to normal activities within a day. Whether or not you need a new eyeglass prescription after surgery will depend on how well you see with your new intraocular lens. If the newly implanted lens doesn't take care of your vision correction adequately, you will need eyeglasses. Your doctor will likely give you a temporary pair until you get your prescription filled.

Who Covers the Costs for Cataract Surgery?

Medicare and private insurance cover costs only for standard cataract surgery that typically includes a single focus lens, usually for distance. Although you'll likely need to wear eyeglasses afterward to accommodate near vision and possibly astigmatism, you won't have out-of-pocket costs. However, if you choose a premium intraocular lens offering additional features, you'll be responsible for any additional costs. Those fees also include the use of the newest high-tech instruments to ensure the selection of the correct lens power and possibly a laser procedure.

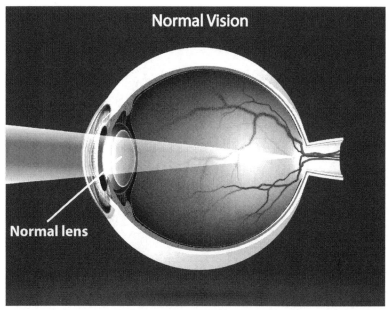

Normal Vision

Normal lens

In a normal eye, light passes through the lens directly to the retina. The image seen is sharply focused.

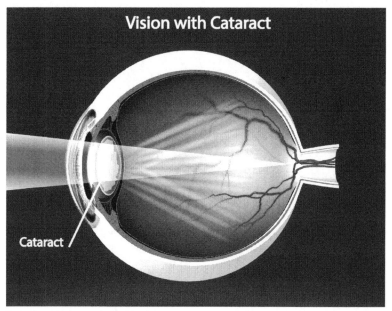

Vision with Cataract

Cataract

Notice how the lens is clouded by the cataract. Incoming light is scattered when it reaches the retina, and vision is distorted.

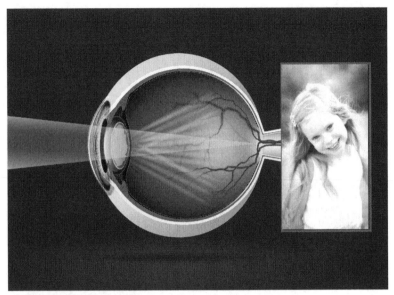

One of the symptoms of cataracts is seeing colors as faded or with a yellowish cast.

| **Normal Vision** | **Vision with Cataract** |

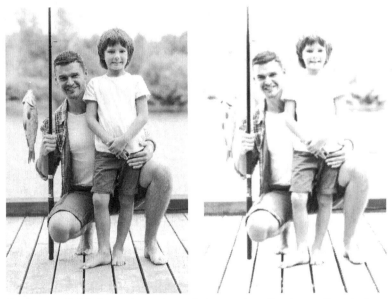

The photo on the left shows colors as seen with the normal eye. The photo on the right shows colors as they may appear with a cataract.

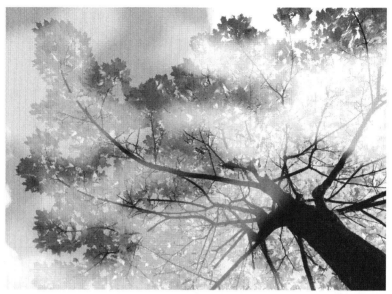

Some individuals with cataracts describe their vision as being cloudy, blurry, or foggy as shown in the example above.

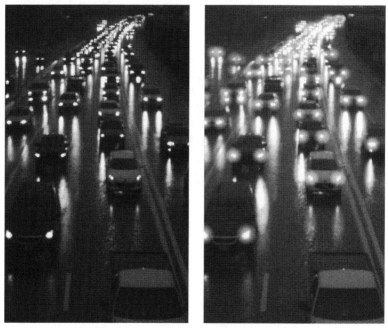

Another common symptom of cataracts is glare—it may occur when you're in sunlight. It may also occur at night. For example, you may see glare in the form of "halos" around lights in traffic.

Basic Steps of Cataract Surgery

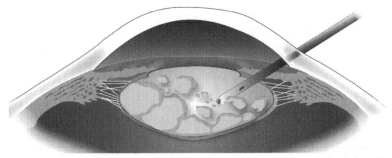

With the phacoemulsification technique, a vibrating probe is inserted into the cloudy lens. The probe breaks the lens into tiny pieces, and they are suctioned out.

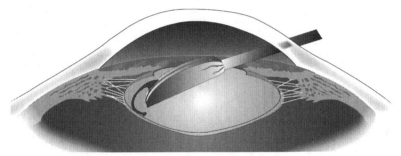

After the cataract has been removed, a new intraocular lens is inserted. The lens is folded when inserted; it then unfolds.

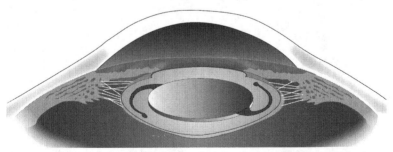

The new intraocular lens is in place. The struts, or "arms" on the sides of the lens, hold it in place.

5

Undergoing Cataract Surgery

As stated earlier, cataract surgery is the most common surgical performed today. More than 3 million Americans undergo the procedure each year, and the
vast majority of them are happy with the results. With
today's surgical techniques and high-tech equipment, removing a cataract and inserting a new intraocular lens can
be completed quickly and efficiently depending on your
needs. But what can you expect from the procedure? This
chapter describes what occurs before, during, and after
cataract surgery.

Prior to Surgery

Cataract surgery is usually performed in an outpatient
surgical center. To ensure patient safety, these centers
must meet strict certification and licensing standards.
Prior to the day of your surgery, your doctor's nursing
staff will give you instructions for arriving at the surgery
center. Even though the procedure may take between ten
to sixty minutes, expect to be at the outpatient center for
up to two hours. You'll have a short recovery period after
the surgery, but most of the time will be spent preparing
you for the procedure. Actually, your preparation begins
before you arrive at the outpatient center; there are
several things you need to know and do in preparation
for cataract surgery.

Using Eye Drops

Because infection is a serious potential problem with eye surgery, you'll likely be asked to apply special eye drops several times a day in the days leading up to your procedure and for several weeks afterward. Doctors usually order *antibiotic* or *antibacterial* drops to destroy or slow the growth of germs that may cause severe eye complications. *Steroidal anti-inflammatory* eye drops are also used to decrease any discomfort and light sensitivity and to promote healing. However, some doctors are performing cataract surgery that does not require eye drops.

Whatever your doctor recommends, it's important that you follow instructions precisely so you experience the full benefits. You'll likely have to apply one drop of each medication several times a day, waiting a few minutes between applications. If you're having difficulty inserting the drops, it may help to have a family member or friend help you. In either case, the best way to make sure the drops make contact with your eyeball is to tilt your head back or lie down.

Because the natural reflex of your eye is to blink to avoid any object, including eye drops, it may take practice to ensure that each eye drop lands squarely on the surface of the eye or inside the pink layer of the inner lower eyelid. If an eye drop medication falls on your eyelashes or outer eyelid, you'll have to try again. Don't be worried if you accidentally apply several drops—they won't hurt your eye. After applying the medication, it's important not to blink for a minute or so because blinking pushes the drops from the surface of the eye into the tear ducts. After applying the drops, gently close the eye without squeezing the lid and hold it shut for at least a minute so the drop can spread across the surface and penetrate into the cornea. Be sure to wash your hands before applying eye drops.

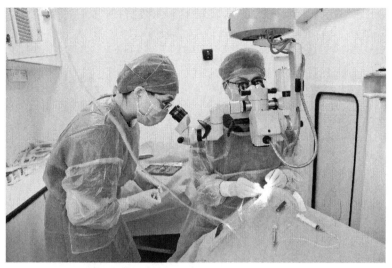

Cataract surgery is performed under a microscope. Removal of one cataract usually takes ten to fifteen minutes, but some procedures may take an hour.

Food and Drug Intake

Your eye surgeon will give you instructions about what you can eat or drink the day of your surgery. You'll likely need to fast or avoid solid foods for at least six hours prior to the procedure, even though you can drink clear liquids for up to two hours prior to the surgery. You also can take your regular medications with sips of water.

There are exceptions to taking your medications, however. If you're diabetic and taking insulin, for instance, you may be asked to stop your medication until after the procedure. Taking oral or injectable insulin at the same time you're fasting can cause your blood sugar to drop to unsafe levels, so you'll likely need to wait to take a drug such as insulin until after surgery. Your doctor may even schedule your procedure immediately in the morning so you can resume your medications and diet quickly.

If you take other medications, such as nitroglycerin pills, or use an inhaler, you'll need to take them with you to the surgery center. Because there's little risk of excess bleeding with today's topical anesthetic and cataract surgical techniques, you likely won't have to stop taking blood thinners, such as *Coumadin (warfarin),* for weeks prior to surgery. Because the small-incision surgery is performed with no sutures and without anesthetic injections, you're unlikely to be at risk for bleeding.

Before Leaving Home

Your doctor and his or her nursing staff will give you a list of instructions before you go home after surgery. But there are a few things you can do on your own prior to your scheduled surgery to ensure a safe and comfortable experience.

- *Arrange a ride home.* Because the pupils of your eyes will be dilated, you won't be able to drive yourself home. The nursing staff won't discharge you unless you have someone designated to pick you up after your procedure. It's important to ask a friend or family member in advance. Also, it's not recommended that you take a cab home because a cabdriver won't be able to stay with you if you should be having any problem upon arriving at your home.

- *Organize your insurance information.* Even though you've likely presented your insurance cards and other documentation during previous doctor appointments, the surgical staff will no doubt ask to see any relevant paperwork again so make sure you have it with you.

- *Dress for surgery.* Cataract surgery doesn't require a hospital gown, but you'll still want to wear comfortable, loose clothing. Because you'll be laying down for the procedure, the best options may be slacks and a short-sleeve shirt or blouse for easy access to your arm or upper chest. Do not wear eye makeup or other facial makeup, and leave your jewelry and other valuables at home.

Preoperative Preparations

When you arrive at the outpatient center for your procedure, your doctor will review your pre-surgical tests and any special instructions. You'll undergo several last-minute preoperative steps. They will likely involve:

- *Position for surgery.* To ensure that you're relaxed and perfectly still during your procedure, you'll be asked to lie on your back with pillows and blankets making you comfortable. Sterile cloth will be draped over your head and shoulders, leaving only your eye exposed.

- *Vital signs.* You'll also be hooked up to various monitors so your anesthesiologist or nurse anes-thetist can monitor your blood pressure, heart rate, and oxygen saturation during the procedure. You will receive oxygen through a tube that fits into your nostrils or you may be in an "oxygen tent" covered by the drape.

  You may even undergo an *electrocardiogram* or *EKG* to monitor the electrical activity of your heart. If your initial vital signs should be unstable, your doctor will likely cancel the procedure and may even send you to the emergency room to avert a health crisis.

- *Anti-anxiety medication.* Most people are anxious about having surgery on their eye. If your anxiety level is high or you are prone to panic attacks, your doctor may give you anti-anxiety medication prior to your procedure. *Valium (diazepam),* for instance, is a drug commonly given for anxiety before surgery. An anti-anxiety drug is usually administered orally shortly before surgery so it's in your system just long enough to make you calm. Anti-anxiety medications are usually very safe, especially when taken only once before surgery.

- *Intravenous (IV) preparation for light sedation.* Whatever your level of anxiety, doctors often order light sedation to keep patients relaxed throughout the procedure. The most common medications used for IV sedation are drugs such as Versed *(midazolam)* that work by slowing the central nervous system. If you're undergoing intravenous sedation, your doctor will insert a very thin needle, attached to a tiny plastic tubing called an *indwelling catheter* or *cannula* into the back of your hand or inside the elbow of your arm. When the needle is removed, the tubing remains until after surgery. The medicine is administered in small amounts.

Receiving Anesthesia

Your surgical team will likely include a board-certified anesthesiologist or certified registered nurse anesthetist, whose role is to make you safe and pain-free by monitoring you throughout the procedure. Your eye surgeon has several options for numbing your eye prior to the procedure. General anesthesia, or putting you to sleep, is rarely used for cataract surgery, unless you have other health issues or severe anxiety that call for it. Otherwise, your doctor will likely recommend local or topical anesthesia, both of which are safe and effective.

Topical Anesthesia

Cataract surgery is performed most often with *topical anesthesia*—anesthetic drops to the eye. These drops block sensation, but don't affect your general consciousness. Topical anesthesia is considered the safest approach possible because no needles are injected into the eye area. Drops or gel are applied to the surface of the eye to numb it. The eye is still capable of moving but you don't feel anything. Your doctor may enhance the drops with intravenous sedation to relax you. You'll still be awake, but may feel drowsy and have only a "foggy" memory about the procedure afterward. One disadvantage of topical anesthesia is that it may allow for unexpected movement of the patient's eye; however, the advantage of topical anesthesia is that does not create stress on the body.

Local Anesthesia

Cataract surgery can also be performed with *local* or *regional anesthetic,* meaning an anesthetic solution is injected into or around the eyeball, eliminating any discomfort. With one method, the surgeon injects a needle through the lower eyelid to an area behind the eye to both numb the eye as well as make the muscles that move the eye immobile. A second regional anesthesia approach involves injecting two or three areas on the side of the eye with an anesthetic. The benefits of both of these approaches are that the eye can't move unexpectedly during surgery. It's also so numb that there's no chance for any discomfort.

Because of the increased risk of eye damage, however, these injections are rarely used today. The exceptions may be in the case of extremely dense cataracts or a very anxious patient. The needle may injure the optic nerve or other sensitive structures around the eye. It may also cause bleeding that can lead to complications after surgery. For instance, you can sustain a temporary bruised or black eye. For these reasons, topical anesthesia has largely replaced injections for cataract surgery since the early 1990s.

Opening Your Eye for Surgery

Successful and safe cataract surgery depends on how well your doctor can see inside your eye. Even with today's effective surgical techniques, your ophthalmologist still needs to view all regions of your eye clearly to work effectively and safely. He or she has various techniques to ensure both.

Dilating Your Pupils

The size of your pupil, or the center opening of the eye that lets in light, is the most important factor for safe and successful cataract surgery. Because removing your lens and replacing it with an intraocular lens takes place behind this portion of the eye, it's imperative that the pupil be as open or dilated as much as possible. You're at higher risk for complications if your surgeon has to work through a small or constricted pupil rather than a enlarged opening that offers a clear view inside your eye.

Before your surgery, your doctor or nurse will apply special dilation drops. He or she may use a medication-soaked sponge or pad of sterile gauze, called a *pledget,* to open the pupil. Studies have shown this approach to be safe and effective as well as comfortable and convenient. In either case, the drugs enlarge the pupil in one of two ways: They either temporarily paralyze the *iris sphincter,* the muscle that makes your pupil larger and smaller, so it won't narrow; or they stimulate the iris to simply remain open. If you have light eyes (blue, green, or hazel), your pupils will likely be more sensitive to the drops so they dilate faster than darker eyes.

Depending on which medication your surgeon chooses, your pupil will remain dilated from three hours to a day, and perhaps longer. Your doctor will also apply antibiotic and anti-inflammatory drops.

Gaining Access to Your Eye

Your doctor will use a medical device, called a *speculum,* to keep your eyelids open during surgery. A speculum allows your physician to work without worrying that your eye will close reflexively. Made of lightweight materials that ensure comfort, some speculums are as simple as wire braces. Others have adjustable, angled arms. While your eye is being held open, the medical staff will apply moisturizing eye drops throughout the procedure to keep your eyeball from drying.

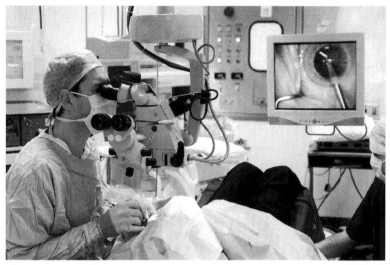

After removing a cataract, an ophthalmologist inserts a folded intraocular lens through an incision about one-eighth inch long. After insertion, the lens unfolds.

Magnifying Your Eye

Because the eye is extremely delicate, performing surgery on it requires that the surgeon has the ability to clearly see all the eye tissue. Doctors once relied on magnifying eyeglasses to work inside the eyes, but today's *ophthalmic surgical microscopes* offer unprecedented detailed images of every region and structure of the eye. Equipped with binocular-type eyepieces and various lighting options, a surgeon can perform precision work within the smallest of areas. Using a foot pedal, an eye surgeon can adjust the magnification of the microscope, and a tiny camera also projects pictures of the patient's eye on a television monitor. The ophthalmic microscope is a critical tool in performing cataract surgery safely.

Cataract Removal

Most cataract surgeries today are performed with a procedure called *extracapsular cataract extraction*. The medical terminology may sound complicated, but it simply means that your surgeon removes the lens of the eye from the transparent membrane or *capsule* that completely surrounds it. He or she then inserts a new intraocular lens into the capsule. This procedure is often referred to as *small-incision surgery,* in part because the development of the foldable intraocular lens allows doctors to reduce the length of the incision necessary to work safely within the eye. Ophthalmologists no longer needed a six- to ten-millimeter incision to remove a cataract and insert a new lens—they can perform the procedure through approximately a three-millimeter incision.

Phacoemulsification

A major refinement to cataract surgery is a technique called *phacoemulsification.* Today, nearly 95 percent of all cataract surgeries are performed with this approach. The eye surgeon makes a short incision in the cornea, where there are no blood vessels. He or she then exposes the front of the lens with a small circular tear, made manually. (If using a laser, the ophthalmologist will make a tiny incision with the laser beam, rather than make a tear.) Then, the ophthalmologist inserts a vibrating *ultrasound probe.* This probe delivers sound waves in a rapid, circular, back-and-forth motion until the hard core of the cataract is *emulsified* or broken into pieces. The tiny pieces can then be suctioned from the eye with the probe's vacuum.

After the cloudy lens is removed, a foldable, artificial lens is inserted into the *posterior capsule*—the remaining back portion of the pocket. The new lens unfolds into position where the old, natural lens once sat. The surgeon positions it with micro-instruments.

Phacoemulsification offers many advantages for patients. Because the incision is only two to three millimeters, individuals are usually able to undergo cataract surgery with topical anesthetic eye drops or a local anesthetic, rather than forms of anesthesia that put you to sleep. Furthermore, they're less likely to develop astigmatism

Phacoemulsification

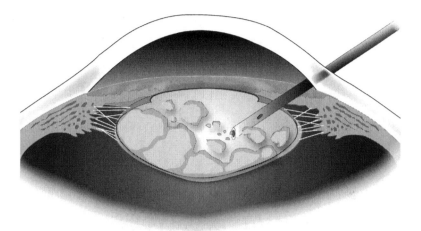

The newer technique, phacoemulsification, eliminates the need for the larger incision once used for cataract removal. The tiny probe shown above vibrates rapidly in a circular, back-and-forth motion, breaking up the old lens (with the cataract) and then removes the pieces with suction.

(blurred vision from corneal irregularities) than with other approaches.

The smaller incision also eliminates or reduces the need for stitches after the intraocular lens is in place. The incision virtually seals itself. Because of this, phacoemulsification is often referred to as a "no-stitch" procedure. The doctor applies a plastic shield to protect the eye as it heals. Individuals usually resume normal activities the next day. Typically there are no restrictions.

Phacoemulsification also provides a benefit to ophthalmologists. Even though it is considered technically difficult to learn and requires expensive, high-tech equipment to perform, doctors can remove a cataract and insert a replacement lens in a safer and more efficient manner.

Conventional Extracapsular Cataract Extraction

Even though phacoemulsification has largely replaced older methods for cataract removal, your doctor may still suggest the older, large-incision method. It is called *extracapsular cataract extraction,* and was once the standard surgical technique. No vibrating probe is used.

With this older approach, the surgeon makes a ten-millimeter incision in the front of the lens and then applies pressure with special instruments on the nucleus of the lens to remove it. Soft material is then suctioned out before a special plastic material is injected into the capsule to keep it in shape while a new lens is positioned. Unlike phacoemulsification, conventional surgery requires several stitches. Even though healing can take several months, you usually can carry out sedentary activities within one or two days after surgery. However, you're likely to have initial restrictions, such as not bending, lifting, or stooping for at least a month.

Because this surgery doesn't involve the constant vibration on the cornea, it may be used for removing advanced or very hard cataracts. It also may be used when someone has other eye problems that could be aggravated by phacoemulsification.

Intracapsular Cataract Surgery

Cataract surgery can also be performed with another approach called *intracapsular cataract extraction.* This method is also sometimes referred to as a *large-incision surgery* because the doctor makes a five-eighths-of-an-inch incision, about half the circumference of the cornea, to enter the eye. He or she then injects medicine to dissolve the fibers, holding the capsule in place. A special *cryoprobe* is then applied to freeze the cataract. As the probe is withdrawn, the lens *and* lens capsule come with it. The doctor implants an intraocular lens in front of the colored iris before stitching the incision closed with tiny sutures.

Large-Incision Surgery

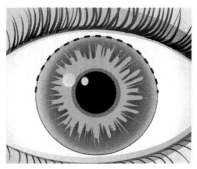

Although the initial incision to enter the eye is longer with intracapsular cataract extraction than previously described procedures, the real distinction with this method is that both the natural lens *and* capsule are removed. As a result, the pocket for the intraocular lens no longer exists. Accordingly, the lens is implanted in front of the iris, rather than behind it.

The technique known as *large-incision surgery* is used when an ophthalmologist believes there is risk of damage to eye tissues from the vibration of the phacoemulsification probe. Here, and incision, about five-eighths of an inch is made to remove the cataract.

This large-incision technique is still used in countries that don't have the skilled specialists or operating room microscopes and other high-technology equipment needed to perform phacoemulsification. However, its appeal is limited in more-developed countries because of long recovery periods and high complication rates, particularly involving astigmatism.

Laser Cataract Surgery

Laser cataract surgery relies on a high-intensity light beam to perform some of the most critical and challenging steps in removing a cataract with phacoemulsification. The laser replaces traditional handheld, diamond-blade cutting tools and lessens the reliance on the ultrasound probe used with phacoemulsification.

The key to such precision is an automated instrument, called a *femtosecond laser,* that replaces metal and diamond blades for making the initial incision in cataract surgery. The laser emits ultrafast infrared pulses, each one lasting a quadrillionth of a second. Because the laser is computer controlled, it can be programmed to at-

Implanted Lens

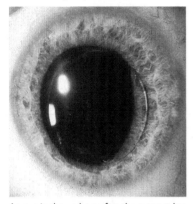

An eye is shown here after the cataract has been removed and the intraocular lens has been inserted. © *2015 American Academy of Ophthalmology*

tain exacting results not attainable with other surgical methods. The surgeon creates a precise surgical plan with sophisticated three-dimensional imaging called *optical coherenece tomography (OCT)*.

Using the laser, the doctor then makes a near-perfect incision on the edge of the cornea, which means there may be less chance of the incision being burned or distorted. The surgeon can also create a very precise circular opening in front of the cataract, which helps position it for removal. Furthermore, the laser pulses soften the cataract, reducing the amount of ultrasound energy needed to break up the lens and suction it out. Even though phacoemulsification is very safe, the laser lessens the chance of vibrations from the probe damaging the sensitive cornea and affecting vision.

If you have astigmatism (blurred vision), your doctor can also perform a second procedure during your cataract procedure. Using the laser, the doctor can make incisions at opposite edges of the cornea to correct the astigmatism. Called *limbal relaxing incisions,* these incisions cause a flattening of the steep cornea, which makes it more round and changes the way light hits the retina. So, not only is the cataract treated, but the astigmatism is surgically corrected. The laser has other benefits, too. By using the laser, your doctor can center your intraocular lens more precisely, which results in better vision. And, because the incision is so exact, the risk of infection after surgery is reduced and healing improves.

Medicare and private insurance don't cover use of the laser for cataract surgery, so it's not usually used in a standard procedure. Yet for individuals who want premium lenses or correction for astigmatism, leading ophthalmologists believe that the laser produces superior results.

Treatment for Cataracts in Both Eyes

If you have a cataract in one eye, you're likely to develop one in the other eye. Most people with age-related cataracts, in particular, eventually experience clouding in the second eye. Cataracts can develop at different rates, but they also can grow at the same rate. If you have cataracts that need to be removed from both eyes, your doctor will decide which one to address first. Surgery is not performed on both eyes at once. Your surgeon will likely remove the worst cataract first and wait a week or two before removing the second cataract, allowing time for the first eye to heal; the exception to this would be if the vision is so different in each eye that it causes an individual problems with balance and judging depth. Also, your insurance company may have guidelines related to how soon your coverage will pay for a second procedure on the second eye.

After Your Surgery

After your surgery, you'll be in a recovery room for about fifteen minutes or more just to make sure that your vital signs are stable and there's no immediate problem from the surgery. You'll also be given eye care instructions. Your eye will likely be covered with a transparent protective shield that you'll be asked to wear for one to several days.

Your doctor will also explain any symptoms that you need to report promptly. Severe eye pain or diminished vision may indicate a complication that needs to be addressed immediately. Finally, you'll be scheduled for your first postsurgical checkup in a day or two after the surgery. Some doctors are doing the postoperative exam later the same day.

6

Recovering from Cataract Surgery

Most people recover very well and very quickly from cataract surgery. Still, removing your cataract and inserting an intraocular lens carries with it some normal short-term and longer-term side effects as well as potential complications. Although the strong likelihood is that you'll be back to your normal activities within days, it is important to follow your ophthalmologist's instructions for recovering from cataract surgery.

Success Rates with Cataract Surgery

Cataract surgery is one of the safest and best-tolerated procedures in medicine. Most patients recover quickly and do very well long term. Overall success rates are between 85 and 92 percent, with some eye surgeons experiencing even higher rates among their patients. The vast majority of cataract surgeries—some statistics suggest as high as 98 percent—are performed without serious complications. Ninety-five percent of individuals experience substantially improved vision. They report both restored visual acuity and better color perception. In fact, some report the best vision they've experienced in years.

There are several reasons for high patient satisfaction. The techniques and technology associated with phacoemulsification and IOLs have reduced the risk of blindness and other serious complications associated with other cataract removal approaches and eliminated the need for thick glasses. Topical anesthesia has eliminated the complications of general anesthesia and anesthesia by injection often used in past operations. Finally, improved antibiotics are enabling physicians to prevent and combat debilitating infections.

Because recovery from cataract surgery differs among individuals, it's important not to compare your experience with others. The length and success of your recovery will depend, in part, on the skills and technique of your eye surgeon along with your own eye and general health.

Common Side Effects of Cataract Surgery

No matter how successful your cataract surgery, you may experience normal side effects as your eye begins to heal. Fortunately, the great majority of symptoms after the procedure are mild, temporary, and easily resolved.

Clouding or Blurriness

These are normal side effects as your eye adjusts to your cataract being removed and your natural lens being replaced. Many patients have clear vision just hours after surgery while others take two to four weeks to see clearly. In either case, cloudy vision eventually disappears in most cases.

Light Sensitivity

Removing a cloudy natural lens and replacing it with one that no longer blocks light sometimes requires an adjustment. For several weeks or even months, you may be very sensitive to bright light. You may experience the same sensitivity if you have any residual postoperation inflammation in your eye. This sensitivity should subside over time. It's especially important to wear sunglasses when you're outside because you no longer have a cataract that blocks light.

Gritty Sensation

Feeling like you have sand in your eye sometimes occurs because your eyelids were open during surgery, causing the eyeball to dry out. Even though a surgical assistant continually lubricates the eye surface with a balanced salt solution during surgery, dry spots may occur afterward. These spots eventually heal, reducing the gritty sensation. It is okay to use artificial tears during the postoperative period.

Floaters

During recovery you may notice tiny specs in your vision. These "floaters" are usually harmless and don't produce any long-term problems; however, because persistent floaters can be a symptom of a more serious issue, such as retinal detachment, you should report to your doctor that you're having them.

Potential Complications of Cataract Surgery

Even though cataract surgery generally produces excellent results, it's not risk-free, especially if you have other eye problems. Diseases such as macular degeneration and glaucoma can make the cataract surgery more difficult to perform, with outcomes that aren't always as good as those in a healthy eye.

Complications can occur during surgery, within a few days or weeks following surgery or even months after recovery. That's why it's important to report any symptoms, such as severe pain, sudden vision loss, seeing flashing lights, or having excessive discharge. Even though serious problems with cataract surgery are rare, inform your doctor about any such symptoms.

Short-Term Complications

Some short-term complications associated with cataract surgery could occur within the first few hours or days after your actual procedure. They may include:

Endophthalmitis or inner eye infection. Infection after cataract surgery is exceedingly rare. Yet it can be damaging if it advances to an infection of the inner eyelid, a condition called *endophthalmitis.* The infection can cause a variety of symptoms, from reddened and swollen eyes to severe pain and diminished or even lost vision. Your doctor will take every precaution to prevent infection, including the application of antibiotic drops before, during, and after surgery. Some surgeons are performing surgery that does not require the use of eye drops in the days following surgery; instead, they insert medication in the eye at the end of the procedure. However, if you are applying eye drops at home, it is important that you follow your doctor's instructions carefully.

Bleeding. Bleeding from cataract surgery, is rare, but can occur. Your doctor works through a tiny incision in a clear portion of the cornea that has no blood vessels, limiting the possibility of bleeding. However, the iris has blood vessels and can bleed. If this occurs, your doctor can simply *cauterize* or seal the spot to stop any bleeding. The back of the eye is not involved, so bleeding from this area is exceedingly rare.

Leaking wound. The vast majority of patients undergoing cataract surgery with today's techniques experience no problems with their incision. It's usually self-sealing, meaning that the natural internal pressure of the eye holds the incision tightly closed, allowing the cornea to heal. At times, however, the incision doesn't heal properly, which allows leaking that can lead to infection. If that occurs, your doctor may place a tiny suture or pressure bandage on the area to help it seal.

Rupture of the posterior capsule. Your eye surgeon will make every attempt to maintain the integrity of the capsular bag (membrane) so it can hold and correctly position your intraocular lens. But because the bag is extremely thin, it can rupture or tear during your surgery;

the success of the procedure depends on the skill of the surgeon, and the surgeons' rates range from 0.1 percent to 10 percent. Unfortunately, such a rupture cannot be repaired, so the ophthalmologist needs to have a plan to deal with this potential complication. If a rupture should occur, the ophthalmologist may need to perform a more complicated operation that involves removing the vitreous gel in the center of the eyeball, and placing the intraocular lens one millimeter in front of the area where it would usually sit. This approach is not a surgeon's preference, but it can still produce a good result for the patient.

Retinal detachment. Another unusual complication of cataract surgery, a retinal detachment can be a problem if you're extremely nearsighted. With this condition, your retina pulls away from the underlying tissue, causing a break or complete tear of the retina. Your symptoms may include seeing floaters and what appear to be flashing lights. You may also have the sensation of a curtain or veil being pulled over your eyes. If you have *any* of these symptoms, you need to report them to your cataract surgeon immediately. Delayed treatment can lead to permanent tissue damage in your eye. A retinal detachment is a medical emergency that should be treated immediately. With prompt treatment, the overall prognosis is usually good.

Secondary glaucoma. An increase in eye pressure after cataract surgery, this condition is unusual. Yet you may be at risk for developing it if you have bleeding or other inflammation. Increased eye pressure causes blurring and aching around the eye; it may also cause nausea. Fortunately, secondary glaucoma is usually temporary. Depending on the extent of your symptoms, your doctor may order eye drops or even perform a laser treatment on your eye to relieve the fluid and lower the pressure.

Astigmatism. A distortion of your cornea during surgery often occurs if your cornea swells or if your eye surgeon has closed the incision with sutures or stitches. After the swelling has subsided or the stitches have been removed, your cornea should return to its original shape, depending on the size of the incision. Smaller is better.

Long-Term Complications

Although most cataract surgery complications occur within the first week after the surgery, other complications may surface well into your recovery.

Dislocated intraocular lens. Even though intraocular lenses are usually held securely in place by the posterior capsule, sometimes they move slightly. The slippage is usually due to weakness in the fibers, or zonules, holding the membrane in place. It can also be caused by conditions such as *pseudoexfoliation* (dandruff-like flakes on the eye's surface), *Marfan's syndrome* (a genetic disorder that affects the body's connective tissues), and *homoscytinuria* (an inherited problem with metabolizing amino acids). Slippage of an intraocular lens is rare. If the lens is still positioned centrally and not interfering with your vision, your doctor likely won't suggest corrective surgery. But if it's causing symptoms, such as faded or double vision, halos, glare, or images that appear to be shimmering, your eye surgeon may need to remove and reposition the lens.

Swelling of the macula. During the first months after surgery, it is possible to experience swelling or *edema* of the macula, the tissue in the center of your retina. Such swelling is caused by a temporary buildup of fluid. Because the macula is crucial to your vision, the swelling may cause blurred vision. Even though this swelling usually resolves on its own, your doctor may prescribe a course of anti-inflammatory eye drops as treatment.

Swelling of the cornea. After cataract surgery, fluid sometimes accumulates in the cornea, the clear window at the front of your eye. The buildup can cause swelling, which not only blurs vision but can rarely also cause eye pain. Normal swelling is expected after surgery and is usually temporary; it will go away on its own after a few days. But in rare instances, the swelling persists. If this occurs, your surgeon may recommend a *corneal graft procedure* to remove the damaged cornea and replace it with donor tissue.

Secondary Cataract

The most common long-term complication of cataract surgery is *posterior capsular opacification (PCO)* or a thickening and clouding of the thin capsule or membrane that once surrounded your natural lens. Still, this condition is often referred to as a *secondary cataract* or *membrane,* it's really not a cataract at all because once your natural lens was removed your cataract can't come back. This condition can cause gradual, sometimes significant, blurring of your vision.

Instead, the haziness reflects a problem with the capsule holding the lens. During cataract surgery, your doctor makes every attempt to keep the back of the capsule intact after removing the front. The back of the capsule not only stabilizes your new intraocular lens, but also promotes clear vision. Normally this approach works. Still, in 20 to 25 percent of patients, the capsule membrane becomes hazy during recovery. This may occur months after your surgery. Doctors believe the cloudiness occurs because remaining cells from the natural lens have grown into the capsule.

Fortunately, this condition can be remedied with a simple, painless procedure called a *YAG laser capsulotomy.* The procedure involves creating a small opening in the capsule membrane to restore your vision. Before the

YAG Procedure

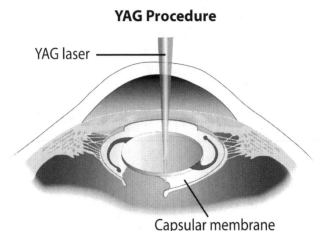

YAG laser

Capsular membrane

Sometimes, after a cataract has been removed, the membrane that holds the intraocular lens will become cloudy. An ophthalmologist can treat this problem with a YAG laser, which makes a tiny hole in the membrane to let light through. The procedure is painless and takes only a few minutes.

procedure, your eye is both numbed and dilated with drops.

The 30-second YAG capsulotomy procedure is performed in the eye doctor's office with a special device called a *YAG laser*. This laser looks much like the slit lamp your doctor uses during your eye exam. While you're looking straight ahead, your ophthalmologist uses the laser beam to remove the hazy posterior capsule; this part of the process takes about thirty seconds. There is no incision and there are no sutures.

Afterward, it may feel like a flashbulb went off in your face. You will be able to drive in five minutes. There are a few risks related to YAG laser treatment. For a few days, you may see what appear to be "gnats" in your vision. They go away quickly.

Other remote risks include nicking the edge of the lens with the laser, which causes no vision issues. As with normal cataract surgery, there's the potential for problems with the retina, even though it's a very rare complication. It is higher in young males with high myopia (highly near-sighted). Even though the possibility of problems is remote, you still need to report seeing flashing lights, increased floaters, or decreased vision to your ophthalmologist immediately.

Your Postoperative Appointment

You'll likely return for an appointment to see your eye doctor a day or two after your cataract surgery. Some ophthalmologists may have you return for a checkup later on the same day of the surgery. During your first postoperative visit, your ophthalmologist will remove the protective shield over your eye and examine your eye to make sure it's healing properly. The doctor will also check your eye pressure and may perform a limited vision exam; however, blurred vision is a common side effect immediately after your surgery.

Because protecting your eye is important, you'll receive instructions about wearing an eye shield while sleeping or napping. You'll also be reminded to wear sunglasses when you're outdoors. Sunglasses will protect your eyes from the sun's ultraviolet rays and also reduce the sensitivity you'll experience to bright light and glare. You will likely be asked to return in one to three weeks for another exam, with other appointments scheduled depending on your progress.

Recovery Guidelines

As mentioned, most individuals who undergo cataract surgery have a quick and relatively trouble-free recovery. You may be advised to rest for the initial twenty-four hours after the procedure and to eat lightly during the first day. But, for the most part, you can return to normal activities immediately thanks to today's improved surgical techniques. Even though it will take weeks to months for your eye to completely heal, you can resume work, hobbies, exercise, and even driving after the first day.

Still, you're urged to follow these instructions during the first week after your surgery:

Limit Strenuous Physical Activity

Because of today's surgical approaches, you no longer need to refrain from exercise or bending and lifting for weeks after the procedure. However, depending on the surgical technique your doctor used, he or she may still place some restrictions on physical activity. You don't want to engage in any activity that would cause stress for your eye.

Avoid Infection

Because infection can be a serious complication after eye surgery, you'll want to avoid any activity that exposes your eye to dirt, dust, or grime. That means washing your hands before and after using your eye drops and staying out of environments that could increase your risk for infection. (You may have to put off camping in the woods or kayaking down a river until you're completely healed!)

Keep Your Eye Dry

Even though you can bathe and shower in the first few days after surgery, make sure to keep your eye closed to avoid contact with soap and water. This will help you avoid the kind of irritation and bacteria both can cause during healing. Likewise, avoid swimming and hot tubs for at least two weeks.

Remove Discharge Gently

You may experience some initial discharge and itching after surgery; any discharge should be cleared away gently with a tissue. Don't use your fingertips or rub your eye. You can soothe any irritation by applying a warm moist cloth to your eye for short intervals.

Do Not Apply Eye Makeup

Because makeup includes ingredients that can irritate the eye, your doctor may want you to avoid using it during the first few days after your surgery.

Postsurgical Eye Drops

In many cases, you'll be asked to use eye drops for several weeks after your surgery to decrease the risk for infection or inflammation. However, some ophthalmologists are using a newer approach that eliminates the need for the ongoing use of postsurgery eye drops; these doctors are injecting antibiotics and anti-inflammatory drugs into the eye's vitreous gel (the gel-like substance inside the eyeball) at the end of the cataract surgery. With this technique, referred to as *dropless cataract surgery*, the drugs used are time-released and eliminate the need for inserting eye drops during the course of your recovery period.

Using Eye Drops after Surgery

On the other hand, if your ophthalmologist does not use the dropless technique, he or she will usually prescribe multiple eye drops that you'll need to use for several weeks following your surgery. The eye drops include antibiotics to kill any bacteria on the outside of the eye, nonsteroidal anti-inflammatory medication to prevent swelling at the back of the eye, and steroid drops to reduce inflammation and keep you comfortable while your eye heals.

Your doctor will discuss the eye drop regimen, which usually involves inserting the drops two to four times a day over four weeks. You'll also be instructed to allow several minutes between applications so each drug can start to work. When inserting eye drops, remember not to blink, but to close your eyelid carefully after inserting the drops so the medication has a chance to penetrate your eyeball rather than wash into your tear ducts. Your doctor

Eye Drops after Surgery

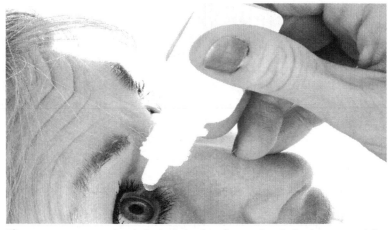

After your surgery, you may be asked to insert eye drops for several weeks. Eye drops prevent infection, swelling, and inflammation.

may also suggest over-the-counter pain relievers if you're having discomfort; he or she may also recommend using artificial tears if your eyes are dry from the surgery. Both the discomfort and the dryness should be only minor problems that will be resolved within days.

Will You Need Eyeglasses after Cataract Surgery?

Whether or not you need eyeglasses after cataract surgery will depend largely on the intraocular lens your doctor implants. Remember, there are two primary goals of cataract surgery: the first is to eliminate the cloudiness by removing your natural lens that has the cataract; the second is to restore clear vision and focusing power with a new intraocular lens.

If you wore eyeglasses before you developed a cataract, you may need them afterward. Because standard monofocal intraocular lenses correct for only one type of vision, usually distance, you likely need prescription eyeglasses for immediate and close-up vision.

If you've selected a multifocal, accommodating, or toric lens, however, you'll significantly reduce or even eliminate your need for eyeglasses. Still, you may need glasses for reading.

In any case, your eye must be completely healed before your doctor prescribes new eyeglasses or contact lenses. Even though many individuals notice a marked improvement in their vision the day after surgery, they usually don't experience the maximum results until several weeks later. By then, the eyes have healed and stabilized enough to be tested for a new eyeglass prescription.

Until you're ready for a new eyeglass prescription, you'll likely be instructed to wear your existing glasses. Even though Medicare Part B doesn't usually pay for eyeglass prescriptions, it does cover the costs of basic framed glasses or contact lenses after cataract surgery. You may incur out-of-pocket fees, however, if you want designer frames or additional features.

The Role of Opticians

Opticians are the technicians who fit you with new eyeglasses or contact lenses, according to the prescription you've received from your eye doctor. Opticians are trained through on-the-job apprenticeships, associate degrees, or certificate programs. Some states require that opticians be licensed and pass certain examinations. Opticians make sure that your new lenses reflect the precise focal power your eye doctor prescribed. Your ophthalmologist will want you to achieve as much visual independence as possible with your intraocular lens. But if you need to supplement the IOL, an optician will help you get the best vision possible with the help of eyeglasses or contact lenses.

Refractive Surgery

You'll recall that our refractive error refers to the type of vision problem we have—be it nearsightedness, farsightedness, astigmatism, or presbyopia. We have these problems because of the way the light bends (or refracts) as visual images hit our retinas. Accordingly, we're prescribed eyeglasses or contacts to correct our "refractive error." However, there are also surgeries, called *refractive surgery,* such as radial keratotomy (RK) and LASIK, that can be performed on your eyes if you don't wish to wear eyeglasses or contacts.

But what if you have had LASIK surgery and later need cataract surgery?

Radial Keratotomy and LASIK

If you have had *radial keratotomy (RK)* or LASIK, you can still have cataract surgery later. Since eye surgeons introduced radial keratotomy in the late 1970s, individuals have undergone this surgery to become less dependent on their eyeglasses by correcting their refractive errors. At one time, radial keratotomy was the most frequently performed surgical technique to correct nearsightedness and astigmatism. It involves using a very thin diamond-cutting blade to make microscopic, spokelike slits in the cornea. As the slits heal, the misshapen areas of the cornea flatten, improving the vision problem. Yet the results are often difficult to predict, and they may change over time and can create problems, such as significant glare.

Since the 1990s, *LASIK (laser in situ keratomileusis)* has replaced radial keratotomy as the most widely performed corneal refractive procedure in the United States. With LASIK, the eye surgeon uses a special laser to improve focusing power by resculpting the cornea at the front of the eyeball. By delivering high-energy pulses of "cool" ultraviolet energy rather than actual heat, the laser can ablate or destroy microscopic amounts of tissue to alter the way light enters the eye and hits the retina. LASIK can flatten the curvature to correct for nearsightedness, steepen the curvature to adjust for farsightedness, or smooth irregular surfaces to restore symmetry altered by astigmatism. Together with high-tech imaging and surgical cutting advances, LASIK produces enhanced safety, effectiveness, and predictability.

What if you have had cataract surgery and want to have LASIK surgery later...is this possible? Most people who have had cataract surgery do not have future LASIK procedures; however, cataract surgery doesn't eliminate the possibility of refractive surgery to permanently correct nearsightedness, farsightedness, or astigmatism. You'll have to wait at least three months after cataract surgery for your eye to heal before subjecting it to another procedure, however. Also, keep in mind that cataract surgery can greatly reduce your dependence on eyeglasses. The premium intraocular lenses available today can reduce your need for—and the expense of—another elective surgery. Talk to your eye surgeon about your options. He or she may suggest a combination surgery called *refractive cataract surgery.*

Refractive Cataract Surgery

Refractive cataract surgery is the term doctors use when merging traditional cataract surgery simultaneously with "refractive" corrections. Here, your doctor doesn't only remove your cataract and insert an intraocular lens. He or she combines sophisticated technology, including a high-tech laser, with premium intraocular lenses to give you optimal vision at all distances; the new lenses also improve astigmatism and presbyopia. You will become less dependent on eyeglasses.

For most individuals, refractive cataract surgery eliminates the need for a separate procedure such as LASIK. Yet your ophthalmologist must make sure that your eye health allows for the combination surgery because it's more aggressive than only removing a cataract and replacing the lens. If you have age-related macular degeneration, for instance, you're not a candidate for refractive surgery. Still, for people who want to reduce dependence on eyeglasses, combining cataract and refractive surgery into one procedure can be beneficial. With refractive cataract surgery, about 95 percent of patients achieve 20/25 or better eyesight without eyeglasses. The other 5 percent can later undergo LASIK to improve vision without glasses.

Commonly Asked Questions

When Can I Drive after Cataract Surgery?

Driving again after cataract surgery depends on when you and your doctor think your vision is clear enough to safely operate a motor vehicle. For some people, that's the next morning. For others, it takes several days or weeks until the swelling subsides and vision clears. There are other considerations that may affect the decision, such as bright lights still bothering you, an old eyeglass prescription that's no longer appropriate, or other eye issues that continue to affect your vision. You'll want to discuss your options with your surgeon. Also, check with your state motor vehicle department to see if there are any restrictions or rules about driving or retesting your vision for your license after cataract surgery.

Can I Wear Contact Lenses with an Intraocular Lens?

If you normally wear contact lenses, you should have no problem wearing them again after cataract surgery. Because your new intraocular lens is positioned in the pocket behind your iris and pupil, it shouldn't interfere with the surface of your cornea where your contact lens sits. As long as you don't have other visual issues or complications that prevent you from using contact lenses, they're an option that your eye doctor will discuss with you. You will, however, need to be retested for a new contacts prescription after your eyes have completely healed.

Is It Possible to Have an Intraocular Lens Implanted if I Didn't Have One with a Previous Cataract Surgery?

Yes, in some rare cases doctors implant an intraocular lens in a separate procedure after cataract surgery. Called a *secondary intraocular lens implant,* it's usually performed because the cataract removal surgery was too complex to safely insert the lens at that time, or there was an injury to the eye. A secondary lens also can be implanted to improve vision in people who had cataracts removed in the past and no longer want to wear the thick glasses or contact lenses they wore in order to see. Whatever the reason, the procedure is similar to that of an initial lens implant.

Should I Wait for Cataract Surgery until There Are Better Intraocular Lenses?

No. If a cataract is significantly impairing your vision you shouldn't wait for the development of a new intraocular lens before considering surgery. Today's options are not only very effective, but they're 99.9 percent safe. That's not to say that medical device companies aren't developing even better options for cataract patients. For instance, even though accommodating lenses are now available, researchers continue to look for improvements so patients have an array of options to achieve complete range of vision. In the meantime, the safety and performance of today's intraocular lenses should far outweigh any concern you might have about having them implanted.

7

Special Conditions and Cataract Surgery

Cataract surgery is considered one of the safest surgical procedures performed today. Yet other eye issues can complicate it. Diabetic retinopathy, glaucoma, high myopia, macular degeneration, or "complicated eyes," for instance, can interfere with your surgery, impact your recovery, and affect your results. Prior to cataract surgery, your ophthalmologist will examine you to check the status of such diseases.

Diabetic Retinopathy

Diabetic retinopathy is one of the most serious complications of both type 1 or type 2 diabetes. It impairs vision by damaging tiny blood vessels in the retinal tissue at the back of the eyeball. According to the National Eye Institute, between 40 and 45 percent of diabetic Americans have some stage of retinopathy, which is also the leading cause of blindness in people with diabetes.

Although diabetic retinopathy is a serious problem on its own, it can also complicate the treatment of cataracts, another common issue for diabetics. The American Diabetes Association estimates that diabetic Americans are 60 percent more likely than other people to develop all types of cataracts. Further, when compared to the general population, they're more likely to develop them at a younger age. Their cataracts also tend to progress at a faster rate.

Types of Diabetic Retinopathy

There are two different types of retinopathy that concern your eye surgeon.

Nonproliferative retinopathy, the earliest and most common form, occurs when the capillaries or tiny blood vessels in the back of the eye balloon into small bulges that leak extra fluid onto the retina. The damage also can result in small spots of blood (*retinal hemorrhages*) and yellow fatty deposits (*exudates*). Even though nonproliferative retinopathy may progress from mild to moderate and finally severe, it doesn't usually require treatment until the macula, at the center of the retina, becomes involved. That occurs when leaking fluid causes the macula to swell until it can't focus properly. This results in blurry central vision.

Proliferative retinopathy is the more serious form of diabetic retinopathy. It progresses over time until the capillaries become so damaged that they close off completely, preventing blood from flowing freely throughout the retina. In response, the retina grows its own new vessels through a process called *neovascularization.* These vessels, however, are so weak that they're also prone to leaking. Instead of supplying proper blood flow to the retina, they cause further damage that can contribute to severe central and peripheral vision loss.

Cataract Surgery with Diabetic Retinopathy

In the absence of retinopathy, the visual outcome for a diabetic after a cataract is removed and replaced should be similar to that of any nondiabetic patient. With retinopathy, however, the outcome will depend on the severity of retinopathy and how well it and your blood glucose levels are controlled.

If you have nonproliferative diabetic retinopathy, for instance, there's a good chance that you can undergo successful cataract surgery without other treatment for your retinopathy. The exception is if your macula is

Diabetic Retinopathy

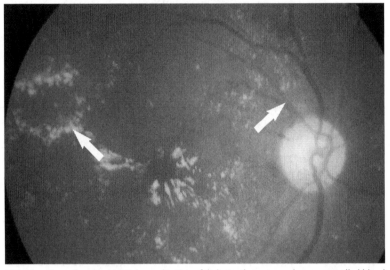

Diabetic retinopathy is a potential complication of diabetes that occurs when uncontrolled blood sugar levels cause damage to the tiny blood vessels of the eye. The arrows above show tiny, abnormal blood vessels; the white spots are fatty deposits, resulting from swelling.

involved. If your condition has advanced to this stage, you may need treatment before cataract surgery. For example, you may have to have a retina specialist perform laser treatment on your retina to stop any leakage.

If you have proliferative retinopathy, you not only have the continued problems of leaking fluid, but other issues as well. Advanced retinopathy can lead to sudden blood bursts (*vitreous hemorrhages*) in the gel center of the eye along with a shrinking of scar tissue that pulls the retina from its normal position (*retinal detachment*). It can also result in a serious type of intraocular pressure buildup (*neovascular glaucoma*) that damages the optic nerve. If you have any of these complications or other signs of significant diabetic retinopathy, your cataract surgeon and retina specialist will need to determine a treatment timetable that safely works with your cataract surgery.

Your eye surgeon will also be conferring with your primary care physician to make sure that you're ready for surgery in terms of your overall health and blood glucose levels. Severely elevated blood sugar, for instance, can raise the risk of infection and poor healing. It can also result in macula swelling that interferes with your achieving the best possible vision.

Glaucoma

Glaucoma is a disease that gradually impairs your peripheral or side vision. It occurs because too much fluid builds inside the eye, causing pressure that can damage the optic nerve. It transmits visual messages from the retina to the brain.

How does this pressure occur? The human eye continually produces clear fluid, called *aqueous humor.* This fluid circulates inside the frontal portion of the eye, behind the iris, through an intricate filtration system. This network of microscopic canals drains the fluid. When the fluid can't drain properly, however, it builds up inside the eye, causing intraocular pressure.

Types of Glaucoma

There are two major types of glaucoma. *Primary open-angle glaucoma,* the most common type, occurs when the drainage system gradually becomes less efficient. Even though the internal pressure in the eyeball is rising, open-angle glaucoma causes no symptoms at first so it's known to "rob" people of their sight before they notice any problem.

A rare form of the disease, *closed-angle glaucoma* (sometimes called *narrow-angle* or *angle-closure glaucoma*) occurs when the iris suddenly and completely (or partially) blocks the eye's drainage angle, the point where the fluid leaves the eye. Patients experience a very fast increase in eye pressure, resulting in sudden vision loss.

Cataracts and glaucoma occur independently of each other. Whether you have open-angle or closed-angle glaucoma, your risk for developing cataracts is about the same as the general population. There are exceptions, however. A secondary condition, such as diabetes, can elevate that risk.

Glaucoma and Cataracts

Having glaucoma should not interfere with cataract surgery. Many aging individuals are treated successfully for both eye problems. Yet glaucoma can have a bearing on the timing of your cataract procedure.

Treating both problems requires a tailored plan that produces the best results with the least risk of continued damage. Your eye doctor will decide on treatment based on the severity of both conditions. If neither disease is interfering with your daily activities, for instance, your ophthalmologist may suggest continuing your pressure-lowering eye drops and monitoring the cataract.

If the clouding starts interfering with your life, however, your eye doctor will need to make choices based on your glaucoma. If it's mild and still successfully controlled, for instance, you'll likely be able to undergo routine and successful cataract surgery, followed by continued treatment for your eye pressure.

If your glaucoma becomes severe, however, your doctor will prioritize treating it versus the cataract. He or she will want to get the pressure under control immediately, especially if it's causing dramatic vision loss because the loss can't be reversed. In fact, your eye doctor may choose to combine cataract surgery with a procedure called a *trabelculectomy,* which is sometimes referred to as *filtration surgery.* The doctor halts the progression of glaucoma by cutting a new pathway to redirect fluid so it bypasses the drainage system section that isn't working properly.

Although ophthalmologists can combine the two procedures, it's done less frequently now than in the past. The most recent scientific findings suggest that glaucoma results are better if the disease is addressed first in a separate operation before removing the cataract. Your eye doctor will base that decision on various factors such as the severity of your glaucoma and the maturity of your cataract.

Cataract surgery can have a beneficial effect on eye pressure, depending on how complicated the surgery is. Today's techniques are believed to improve the pressure inside the eye in many instances. In fact, some statistics suggest that at least 50 percent of glaucoma patients undergoing a relatively simple cataract procedure can experience a several-point decrease in eye pressure. Some patients may not even need eye drops for their glaucoma after cataract surgery.

This reduction in eye pressure, however, varies from person to person. Some individuals with more severe glaucoma likely will need to continue their medication to control the pressure. Also, if your cataract procedure is somewhat complicated, it can actually lead to increased pressure. You may even experience short-term *pressure spikes* after surgery. It's impossible to predict whether your pressure will rise, fall, or stay the same *or* whether any change will be short term or permanent. Your ophthalmologist will explain the possibilities based on your condition.

High Myopia

High myopia is a severe form of nearsightedness—the inability to focus clearly on distant objects. High myopia occurs because one's eyeball has grown significantly in length.

Having a high degree of nearsightedness can slightly increase your risk of developing cataracts sooner than people with normal vision. Because high myopia also can create potential complications with cataract surgery your doctor will take your condition into consideration when planning for your procedure.

The extreme lengthening of the eyeball that can occur with high myopia, for instance, can put you at significant risk for *retinal detachment.* With this condition, the retina stretches, leading to a hole or tear through which fluid can leak. This can cause the retina to detach from the back of the eye, leading to symptoms such as light flashes, "floaters," and a "curtain effect" to your vision.

Many retinal detachments are also associated with *posterior vitreous detachment,* a condition in which the gel in the middle of the eye shrinks and separates from the retina. Although posterior vitreous detachment often occurs as a result of normal aging, it can develop earlier in life if you have severe myopia.

Cataract Surgery with High Myopia

Given the risk of both retinal and vitreous detachment, it's important that your cataract surgeon confers with your retina specialist in preparing for cataract surgery. For instance, because a rupture of the posterior capsule, the pod where your new intraocular lens is placed, can significantly increase the risk of retinal detachment, your doctor must be able to manage such a complication. That not only involves planning for the possibility prior to surgery, but also taking steps during the procedure to deal with the tear, support the capsule, and modify any technique or approach to ensure the intraocular lens is stable.

Age-Related Macular Degeneration

An estimated 10 million Americans suffer from *age-related macular degeneration (ARMD),* a disease that damages the light-sensitive cells of the macula. Because the macula is the part of the eye responsible for central or fine-detail vision, it's no longer easy to read, drive, or do close-up tasks.

Types of Macular Degeneration

Dry macular degeneration is the less serious form of ARMD. It occurs when the macular cells break down slowly, causing a gradual loss of vision. A common early symptom is that straight lines appear crooked or wavy. Because there's no effective treatment for dry macular degeneration, the focus is on good nutrition and taking steps to slow the progression of the disease.

The more serious form of the disease, *wet macular degeneration,* occurs when abnormal blood vessels grow under the macula and leak fluid that damages its tissues. In addition to seeing wavy lines, individuals may also have blurred vision as well as other problems with their central vision. Although there's no treatment to reverse lost vision due to wet macular degeneration, injections to block abnormal vessel growth and laser therapy to stop the leaking can slow the progress. It is critical that anyone with wet macular degeneration see his or her eye doctor immediately upon noticing any changes in vision because permanent damage can occur rapidly.

Age-Related Macular Degeneration and Cataracts

Individuals with macular degeneration have about the same risk for cataracts as the general population. Cataracts develop independently of the disease. They also can be surgically treated despite the presence of either form of the disease. The challenge for your cataract surgeon, however, is to determine the appropriate timing. That means first identifying what part of your vision loss is due to your cataract and what part is due to the macular degeneration.

Macular degeneration can also make a difference in the type of intraocular lens that works best for you. For

Macular Degeneration

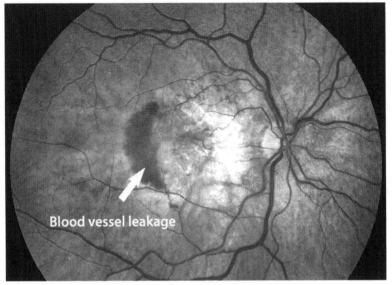

Age-related macular degeneration occurs when the macular, at the center of the retina in the back of the eye, becomes damaged. There are two types of the disease, dry and wet macular degeneration. Wet macular degeneration carries a more serious risk of vision loss.

instance, your doctor likely won't recommend a multifocal lens since it requires normal macular function for success. Also, because the course of macular degeneration varies widely among patients, your cataract surgeon will likely want to work with your retina specialist to tailor the correct plan for treatment.

Complicated Eyes

In addition to common eye diseases that can complicate cataract removal, there are other conditions that may affect your ophthalmologist's recommendation for surgery. If you have one of these conditions, you are said to have *complicated eyes*. That simply means that, although you can undergo cataract surgery, there may be other issues that may pose challenges prior to, during, or after surgery. Your doctor will be alert to them.

Small Pupils

One common type of complicated eyes is a *small pupil*. The size of your pupil, or the opening at the center of your iris, is important in cataract surgery. It must be large enough for your surgeon to work on your lens safely and successfully. Some cataract patients have constricted or small pupils. Even with dilation, not enough light gets into the eye to enable the doctor to perform surgery. Natural aging can cause this problem. But it's also a common side effect of some medications, particularly eye drops prescribed extensively in the past for glaucoma. Long-term use of *pilocarpine* to lower eye pressure, for instance, can permanently restrict the pupils.

Other prescription medications can also cause a weakening of the iris sphincter muscle, referred to as *IFIS* or *intraoperative floppy iris syndrome,* which can also contribute to a smaller pupil. This syndrome was first noted as a side effect of *Flomax (tamsulosin),* an *alpha-adrenergic blocker* used to treat urinary problems in men with enlarged prostate glands. The medication can cause the iris to lose its muscle tone so it can't stay dilated during surgery. Instead, the pupil gets smaller, making it technically more difficult for the eye surgeon to replace the lens. Similar medications for high blood pressure, kidney stones, and urinary tract infections can also result in the same problem.

Whatever the cause, studies show that complications with cataract surgery increase as the pupil shrinks, largely because the shrinkage is blocking the doctor's view. Although a skilled eye surgeon can work through a smaller space, he or she eventually has to use special maneuvers to enlarge the pupil to achieve a safe outcome. The techniques for doing so have improved over the years, so doctors no longer depend on surgically opening the pupil. Today they use special intraocular devices to temporarily stretch and dilate the pupil for surgery. They also have ways to stabilize the iris.

Because of potential small-pupil complications, it's important to provide your cataract surgeon with a complete list of your medications when giving your medical history. If you're taking a drug that may cause intraoperative floppy iris syndrome, your urologist or other specialist may advise you to let your eye surgeon know prior to surgery that you're taking it.

Weak Structures within the Eye

The natural lens of your eye sits in a thin transparent pocketlike structure, called the *capsular bag*. It's suspended behind the iris by thousands of microscopic fibers called *zonules*. When your eye surgeon removes your cataract, he or she places a new intraocular lens in what remains of that pocket. It keeps the lens centered behind the pupil so it provides excellent vision.

In some people, however, the capsular bag and zonules are weakened, making removing and replacing the lens more difficult. It also may increase the risk of complications with cataract surgery. Several factors can cause the weakening, including advancing age plus prior trauma, surgery, or retinopathy involving the eye.

Whatever the cause, a weakened lens capsule and zonules can make cataract surgery technically more demanding than a routine procedure. Performing a thorough dilated eye exam plus taking a complete medical history prior to your operation, however, will help your eye doctor diagnose any potential complications during surgery. Experienced cataract surgeons are prepared to perform various intricate surgical maneuvers and steps to address any of the difficulties that may arise with a weakened lens capsule and zonules. Modern techniques, technology, and tools have greatly improved eye surgeons' ability to deal with these circumstances.

Flaky Deposits on the Eye's Surface

Another special condition that's of concern to your cataract surgeon is *pseudoexfoliation,* sometimes referred to as *exfoliation.* As mentioned earlier, with this disorder, microscopic, whitish flakes, similar to dandruff, are deposited on the front surface of the eye lens as well as the iris, pupil, and drainage meshwork. Although the source of exfoliation isn't fully understood, this condition can cause many eye complications, including those directly related to cataract surgery. For instance, flaking can damage the dilating muscle of your iris, making it more difficult for your eye surgeon to expand your pupil to work safely inside the eye. It can make the lens capsule so fragile that it's prone to tears and ruptures during the procedure.

Pseudoexfoliation can also weaken the zonules holding the capsule in place. In fact, one cataract surgery step that poses a particular risk for complications is *phacoemulsification,* which is performed to break up the cataract. Any pulling, pushing, or putting excessive pressure on the cataract with the phacoemulsification probe may result in the cataract falling to the back of the eye on the retina or optic nerve. It can also prevent the usual stability of a new lens.

Dealing successfully with pseudoexfoliation requires that your eye doctor perform a thorough eye examination prior to surgery so he or she is prepared with the extra tools and for the surgical steps necessary to perform it safely. Because flaking prevents the pupil from dilating well, for instance, special surgical devices, such as *pupil expansion rings,* will be necessary to keep the pupil open fully. Your eye surgeon also will modify his or her surgical maneuvers throughout the procedure to avoid any complications that can cause vision loss. That means taking steps to prevent the capsule from tearing or rupturing or the natural lens from falling into the center of the eyeball. It also involves maneuvering the new intraocular lens in such a way that it's centered and anchored behind the pupil.

In Closing

Cataracts have been impairing vision since the beginning of time. Fortunately, eye doctors today have more effective options than those of physicians centuries ago who simply pushed the lens away from the pupil into the eye's center gel and called it treatment. Needless to say, their primitive attempts, referred to as *couching,* didn't restore sight.

Thanks to modern medicine, cataract treatment today uses sophisticated devices and techniques to remove cataracts safely and restore the best vision possible. With today's intraocular lenses, capable of correcting various vision problems, many individuals can now undergo painless cataract surgery and achieve 20/20 vision without eyeglasses. Even those who still need eyeglasses or contact lenses can experience greatly improved vision.

Whether you need cataract surgery now or in the future, we hope this book has given you the tools you need to find the right eye surgeon, learn about your surgical options, and make good decisions about your cataract treatment.

Resources

American Academy of Ophthalmology
P.O. Box 7424
San Francisco, CA 94120
Phone: (415) 561-8500
www.aao.org

American Optometric Association
243 North Lindbergh Boulevard, 1st Floor
St. Louis, MO 63141-7881
Phone: (800) 365-2219
www.aoa.org

American Society of Cataract and Refractive Surgery and Eye Surgery Education Council
4000 Legato Road, Suite 700
Fairfax, VA 22033
Phone: 703) 591-2220
www.ascrs.org
www.eyesurgeryeducation.org

**The Foundation of the American
Academy of Ophthalmology**
P.O. Box 429098
San Francisco, CA 94142
Phone: (877) 887-6327
www.eyecareamerica.org

National Eye Institute—National Institutes of Health
31 Center Drive MSC 2510
Bethesda, MD 20892
Phone: (301) 496-5248
www.nei.nih.gov

Prevent Blindness
211 West Wacker Drive, Suite 1700
Chicago, IL 60606
Phone: (800) 331-2020
www.preventblindness.org

Glossary

Accommodating IOL: Type of intraocular lens that is designed to move within the eye in order to provide partial focusing ability. Also referred to as an *adaptive* lens.

Anterior capsule: The front of the transparent lens capsular bag through which an opening must be made surgically in order to remove a cataract and implant an IOL.

Anterior chamber IOL: Intraocular lens designed for implantation in front of the iris.

Astigmatism: Refractive error caused by irregular corneal surface scattering light rather than focusing it on the retina; results in blurring at various distances.

Axial length: Distance between the cornea and retina used to determine the correct intraocular lens.

Capsular bag: The transparent membrane surrounding the entire lens of the eyeball.

Cataract: Loss of transparency, or cloudiness, of the natural lens that can impair vision.

Combined procedure: Two separate operations being performed at the same sitting. In the context of cataracts, this usually refers to glaucoma surgery being performed coincident with cataract surgery.

Complicated eye: An eye that has anatomical features that make surgery more difficult.

Conjunctiva: Thin, transparent mucous membrane that overlies the white sclera and lines the inner aspect of the upper and lower lids.

Conjunctivitis: Inflammation of the part of the eye known as the conjunctiva.

Cornea: Transparent, dome-shaped structure at the front of the eyeball through which all light rays enter the eye interior.

Corneal clouding: Vision-impairing loss of corneal transparency.

Cortical cataract: Type of cataract in which a cloudiness is mostly in the regions closest to the front and rear of the lens.

Diabetic retinopathy: Progressive retinal disorder that results from diabetes, causing abnormal growth of tiny blood vessels in the eye.

Dilating drops: Medications given via eye drops to temporarily expand the pupil.

Diopter: Standard optical unit of measure. In the context of eyes, this is the unit for measuring refractive error or the power of prescription eyeglasses.

Dry eye: A lack of surface tear lubrication that typically results in symptoms of minor discomfort.

Dry macular degeneration: A form of macular degeneration in which yellow deposits, called *drusen,* develop in the macula, which is in the center of the retina.

Edema: Swelling.

Extracapsular cataract extraction (ECCE): Type of cataract surgery in which the capsular bag supporting the original lens is preserved in order to hold an intraocular lens.

Femtosecond laser: A laser that replaces metal and diamond blades used for making initial incisions for cataract surgery; named for *femtoseconds,* the laser's pulses last a quadrillionth of a second.

Floater: Moving flecks in the field of vision. The usual cause is age-related liquefaction and clumping of the vitreous gel within the central ocular cavity.

Foldable IOL: Intraocular lens made of silicone or acrylic plastic, allowing it to be folded for insertion through a small cataract incision.

Free radicals: Chemical molecules implicated in damage to tissue. Also referred to as *oxidants* or *oxygen-free radicals.*

General anesthesia: Type of anesthesia in which a patient is unconscious and a breathing tube connected to a respirator is used.

Glossary

Glaucoma: Eye disease caused by prolonged, abnormal elevation of the intraocular fluid pressure.

Halo: Appearance of rings around sources of light, especially at night.

High myopia: Higher-than-average degree of myopia associated with an elongated eyeball.

Hyperopia: Refractive error in which light rays are misrouted behind, rather than on, the retina. Also called farsightedness.

Intracapsular cataract surgery (ICCE): Cataract surgery in which the capsular bag is removed together with the lens.

Intraocular lens (IOL): Artificial lens permanently implanted in the eye.

Intraocular pressure: Internal fluid pressure of the eyeball.

Intraoperative abberometry: State-of-the-art measuring technology that allows surgeons to confirm or revise an intraocular lens power choice in the operating room; makes multiple measurements in less than a minute to determine precise refractive error correction necessary.

Iris: Colored structure located behind the cornea that functions like a curtain to regulate the amount of light that passes to the back of the eye.

Iris sphincter: Circular muscle around the iris that opens and closes the pupil.

LASIK (*Laser in situ keratomileusis*): Refractive surgery that involves laser-guided reshaping of the cornea.

Lens: Transparent intraocular tissue, located behind the pupil, that helps bring rays of light to a focus on the retina.

Local anesthesia: Numbing area around the eye by injecting anesthetic. Sometimes referred to as *regional anesthesia* when injection is made to a specific area such as behind the eyeball (*retrobulbar*) or surrounding the eye (*peribulbar*).

Macula: Circular central-most region of the retina, which produces detailed, fine central vision.

Macular degeneration: Age-related deterioration of the macula, which impairs the central vision.

Macular edema: Clear fluid collecting in the macula, which impairs central vision.

Mature brown cataract: Advanced cataract stage in which the central nucleus becomes solid.

Mature white cataract: Advanced cataract stage in which the lens turns white and becomes totally opaque.

Monofocal IOL: Type of intraocular lens that provides optimal focus without glasses at a single distance.

Monovision: Vision in which two eyes each see at different distances without glasses.

Multifocal IOL: Type of intraocular lens that provides optimal focus without glasses at more than one distance.

Myopia: Refractive error in which light rays are misrouted in front of, rather than on, the retina. Also called nearsightedness.

Nonproliferative diabetic retinopathy: A form of retinopathy characterized by leaky, porous blood vessels in the eyeball.

Nuclear cataract: Type of cataract in which a cloudiness is predominantly in the center region of lens.

Ophthalmologist: Physician specializing in medical and surgical treatment of the eye, including cataracts.

Optic nerve: Nerve that transmits vision from the retina to the brain.

Optician: Eye professional who is licensed to fit and dispense eyeglasses and contact lenses.

Optometrist: Doctor of optometry (OD) who specializing in vision problems, treating vision conditions with glasses, contact lenses, low vision aids, and vision therapy.

Pediatric cataract: Cataract that develops in an infant or child. Often referred to as a *congenital cataract* if present at birth due to genetic or other condition.

Phacoemulsification (Phaco): Surgical technique in which a cataract is ultrasonically broken apart and suctioned from the eyeball.

Pilocarpine: Glaucoma eye drop medication that also constricts the pupil.

Pledget: Small thin sponge that can be placed just beneath the eyelid in order to administer eye medications.

Posterior capsular opacification: Condition in which the posterior capsule becomes cloudy months to years after successful cataract surgery. Also referred to as a *secondary cataract* or a *secondary membrane*.

Posterior capsule: The back part of the transparent lens capsular bag.

Posterior chamber IOL: An intraocular lens designed for implantation behind the iris.

Glossary

Presbyopia: An age-induced refractive error characterized by the inability to focus up close despite clear distant vision.

Proliferative diabetic retinopathy: Form of retinopathy marked by abnormal, new blood vessels growing from the retina into the vitreous.

Pseudoexfoliation: Eye condition characterized by microscopic flakes on the lens as if its capsule were shedding dandruff. Leading cause of glaucoma and complication of cataract surgery. Visible during a dilated-eye examination.

Pupil: Circular opening in the iris through which light passes in order to enter the back of the eye.

Radial keratotomy (RK): Refractive surgical procedure for myopia using radial cuts in the cornea.

Refractive error: Optical imperfection in an otherwise healthy eye that results in blurred vision without glasses at certain distances. Causes nearsightedness, farsightedness, astigmatism, or presbyopia.

Refractive surgery: Surgical procedure to correct refractive errors. Includes *radial keratotomy* and LASIK *(Laser in situ keratomileusis).*

Retina: The thin, light-sensitive tissue that lines the back half of the eyeball and registers vision.

Retinal detachment: Condition in which the retina separates from the inner eye wall.

Sclera: White wall of the eyeball.

Secondary cataract or membrane: Condition in which the posterior capsule becomes cloudy months to years after successful cataract surgery. It's also referred to as *posterior capsular opacification.*

Secondary IOL: An intraocular lens that is inserted during a separate operation subsequent to the original cataract surgery.

Small pupils: Refers to eyes in which the pupil does not dilate normally following insertion of dilating drops.

Snellen chart: Standard eye chart for testing distance vision.

Speculum: Device that holds open the eyelids during eye surgery.

Subcapsular cataract: Type of cataract in which a haze is located adjacent to the front or rear lens capsule.

Tear duct: Microscopic drainage channel for tears located in the corner of the upper and lower eyelid.

Tonometry: Test to measure the internal eye fluid pressure. Can be done via various methods including *noncontact tonometry,* known also as the *air-puff test,* or *Goldmann Applanation Tonometry.* Considered the gold standard, Goldmann produces the most accurate results, in part, because the tonometer's tip touches the eye.

Topical anesthesia: Anesthesia administered via eye drops.

Toric IOL: A special intraocular lens that is designed to reduce higher degrees of preexisting astigmatism.

Trabeculectomy: Surgical procedure for glaucoma, in which a valvelike channel for fluid drainage is created in the eye wall. Also called "filtration surgery."

20/20 vision: Ability to read the rows on an eye chart that correlate with "normal" visual acuity.

Ultrasound: Also referred to as *sonography,* ultrasound uses high-frequency (inaudible) sound waves to develop images inside the eye; works by recording echoes of the waves as they bounce off internal structures, resulting in real-time images relayed on a computer screen.

Ultraviolet (UV) rays: Invisible rays of the sun that have destructive properties. Categorized by wavelength and depth of penetration, UV-A and UV-B both can damage the eye. UV-A rays promote release of damaging *oxidants* or *free radicals* that can lead to the formation of cataracts.

Visual acuity: Quality of central vision.

Vitreous humor: Semisolid, gel-like material that fills the central cavity of the eyeball.

Wet macular degeneration: Form of macular degeneration in which abnormal blood vessels grow under the macular—at the center of the retina.

YAG capsulotomy: Nonsurgical, vision-restoring treatment for a secondary membrane. Relies on special YAG *(yttrium-aluminum garnet)* laser that uses high-intensity light beams to remove the clouded membrane without damaging adjacent tissue.

Zonules: The microscopic ligaments that support the lens and capsular bag.

Index

Index

Index

60–61
for surgery, 44, 59–65
retinal detachment, 71, 86, 90
retinal hemorrhages, 85
retinitis pigmentosa, 10
retinopathy
 diabetic, 9, 16, 50, 84–87
 nonproliferative, 85
 proliferative, 85
retinoscope, 24
Ridley, Harold, 32–33
"ripe" cataracts, 7
risk factors, 9–10, 18
rods, 10
rupture of the posterior
 capsule, 70–71

S

sclera, 25
secondary cataract, 73–75
secondary glaucoma, 71
secondary intraocular lens
 implant, 83
secondary membrane, 73–75
sedation, *see* anesthesia
sharpness of eyes, 19
short-term complications of
 cataract surgery, 69–72
side effects, 68–69
side vision, 19
slit lamp, 26–29
small-incision surgery, 60–61
small pupils, 93–94
smoke/smoking, 10–11
Snellen letter chart, 19–20
special conditions, 84–95
 age-related macular
  degeneration, 90–92
 complicated eyes, 92–95
 diabetic retinopathy, 84–87
 glaucoma, 87–89
 high myopia, 89–90
speculum, 58
steroidal anti-inflammatory
 drops, 52

steroids, 9, 17
subspecialty, 14
success rates, 67–68
sun, 11, 42, 75
sunglasses, 11, 42, 75
surgery
 anesthesia for, 56–57
 anti-anxiety medication for,
  55
 body position for, 55
 for cataracts in both eyes,
  65
 commonly asked questions
  about, 49–50
 complications of, 69–75
 with diabetic retinopathy, 50,
  85–87
 driving after, 82
 dropless, 77
 extracapsular cataract
  extraction during, 59–65
 eye care professionals
  involved in performing,
  45–46
 eyeglasses following, 50,
  78–79
 on eyes, 18
 factors affecting timing of,
  50
 with glaucoma, 50
 insurance coverage for, 50
 intraocular lenses vs., 83
 intravenous preparation for
  light sedation during, 56
 new eyeglass prescriptions
  for avoiding, 49
 planning for, 44–50
 postoperative appointment
  following, 75
 preoperative preparations
  for, 51–56
 recovering from, 65–83
 removing cataracts for, 44
 restrictions following, 50

113

About the Authors

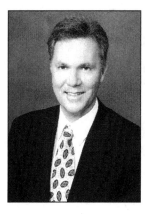

Paul E. Garland, M.D., is an ophthalmologist in private practice at The Eye Center of North Florida, in Panama City. Board-certified in ophthalmology, Dr. Garland specializes in state-of-the-art cataract surgery, performing more than a thousand surgeries annually. He is also trained in *oculoplastic* surgery, in which both cosmetic and reconstructive procedures are performed on the eyelids, tear ducts, and structures within the eye of the eye socket.

Dr. Garland graduated cum laude with a bachelor of arts degree in pre-medicine and economics from Tulane University in New Orleans, Louisiana. He is also a graduate of Tulane University School of Medicine in New Orleans. Dr. Garland completed an internship at Tulane before serving two years as a second lieutenant in the National Health Service Corps. He completed a three-year ophthalmology residency at the University of Utah in Salt Lake City. That residency was followed by a one-year fellowship in oculoplastic and reconstructive surgery at the University of Texas Hermann Eye Center.

Dr. Garland is a member of the American Academy of Ophthalmology, the American Society for Cataract & Refractive Surgery, the Florida Medical Association, and the Bay County Medical Society, among other professional organizations. Dr. Garland may be reached through his website: **www.eyecarenow.com.**

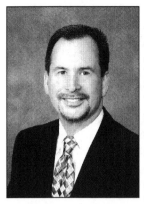

Bret L. Fisher, M.D., is an ophthalmologist in private practice at The Eye Center of North Florida, in Panama City, where he specializes in refractive cataract surgery. Dr. Fisher was the first eye surgeon in Florida to perform femtosecond laser-assisted cataract surgery; he's also skilled in advanced custom LASIK.

A *magnum cum laude* graduate of Duke University, in Durham, North Carolina, Dr. Fisher was also an honors graduate of Duke University School of Medicine. After a general medicine internship at Santa Barbara Cottage Hospital, Santa Barbara, California, he completed his ophthalmology residency at Wills Eye Hospital, Philadelphia, Pennsylvania.

In 1993, Dr. Fisher joined Newberry Eye Clinic in Panama City, Florida, as medical director and attending surgeon. With the merger in 2000 of Newberry Eye Clinic and two other eye practices, Dr. Fisher became the medical director of The Eye Center of North Florida and its freestanding ambulatory surgery center, The Laser and Surgery Center. The Eye Center is nationally recognized for its excellence in performing cataract surgery and the center's ophthalmologists frequently host visiting eye surgeons from around the world.

At The Eye Center of North Florida, Dr. Fisher has also established an active clinical research department. He and his staff have participated in many important studies, including the FDA trials for new multifocal and toric multifocal intraocular lens implants.

Along with coauthor Dr. Garland, Dr. Fisher and staff have also participated in pharmaceutical trials for postcataract inflammation, dry eye, and diabetic eye disease. Dr. Fisher travels widely and frequently lectures on advances in cataract surgery and other ophthalmology issues.

Board-certified by the American Board of Ophthalmology and certified in cataract and implant surgery and LASIK by the American College of Eye Surgeons, as well as being an active member of ASCRS, Dr. Fisher is always up to date on the newest ideas, concepts, and technologies in ophthalmology. He serves as a consultant to the industry and a teacher and mentor to his fellow surgeons.

When he is not working at the clinic or lecturing, Dr. Fisher enjoys spending time at home on his farm with his wife, Katie, and their three children. Dr. Fisher may be reached at: **www.eyecarenow.com.**

Consumer Health Titles from Addicus Books

Visit our online catalog at www.AddicusBooks.com

To Order Books:
Visit us online at: www.AddicusBooks.com
Call toll free: (800) 888-4741

For discounts on bulk purchases, call our Special Sales
Department at (402) 330-7493.
Or email us at: info@Addicus Books.com

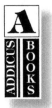

Addicus Books
P. O. Box 45327
Omaha, NE 68145

*Addicus Books is dedicated to publishing consumer health books
that comfort and educate.*